Theatre and Performance in Small Nations

Edited by Steve Blandford

intellect Bristol, UK / Chicago, USA

First published in the UK in 2013 by
Intellect, The Mill, Parnall Road, Fishponds, Bristol, BS16 3JG, UK

First published in the USA in 2013 by
Intellect, The University of Chicago Press, 1427 E. 60th Street,
Chicago, IL 60637, USA

A catalogue record for this book is available from the
British Library.

Cover designer: Holly Rose
Copy-editor: MPS Technologies
Production manager: Jessica Mitchell
Typesetting: Planman Technologies

792.
01
THE

ISBN 978-1-84150-646-3

Printed and bound by Hobbs, UK

Contents

Acknowledgements

This book has been a long time in the making and I would first of all like to thank all the contributors for their patience and persistence. They have all been very supportive as the volume came together and it has been a pleasure working with them throughout.

I would also like to thank Intellect and, in particular, Jessica Mitchell, for her enthusiasm and very efficient handling of the book. It has been a real pleasure to work with them.

The thinking that underpins the book originated in my involvement in the Centre for the Study of Media and Culture in Small Nations at the University of Glamorgan. I would therefore like to thank all my colleagues there for their help and support, particularly David Barlow, the Centre's first Director, Gill Allard, who collaborated with us on the idea of a series of books on media and culture in small nations, and the members of the Centre's steering group, who have provided collegial and scholarly support throughout the period in which the book has been written: Paul Carr, Alice Entwistle, Huw Jones, Ruth McElroy, Stephen Lacey, Lisa Lewis, Philip Mitchell, Ieuan Morris, Catriona Noonan and Rebecca Williams.

Finally, as always, most books are written at the expense of others in one's life and I would like to thank my partner, Mitch Winfield, and my children, Sam and Beth, for their love, encouragement and patience.

Introduction

Steve Blandford

M any commentators have routinely referred to theatre and, to an extent, all forms of
live performance as particularly appropriate to the discussion of national identity.
Put simply, the act of live performance itself draws attention to the idea that
identities are performed and that different versions of identity can compete for our attention
or allegiance.

This collection of chapters from a wide variety of contexts will of course seek primarily to
open up questions regarding the validity of the very category of 'small nation' and the role of
theatre and performance in such contexts. Inevitably, though, it will also add to much wider
debates about nationhood and its construction per se, as Helen Gilbert has put it:

> In the past decade or so, theatre has been increasingly recognised as a critical resource for
> the study of wildly competing discourses about the nation, particularly in countries with
> a history of strong state intervention into cultural practice. Always a site of circulating
> representational forms, theatre becomes, at formative moments in the ongoing narrative
> of nationhood, a means by which communities register, reiterate and/or contest modes
> and models of national belonging.
>
> (Gilbert 2004: vii)

While it would be a distortion to suggest that all small nations have a 'history of strong state
intervention into cultural practices', it is nevertheless legitimate to claim that the idea of
small nationhood is inevitably bound up with questions of power and that the majority of
small nations are, or have been, involved in contested definitions of identity of a particularly
intense nature. Frequently, especially in cases where nationhood does not bring with it the
full power of the state, cultural practice becomes a crucial site where such contested
definitions are played out.

A clear example can be found in a powerful case that is not represented in this volume,
but is nevertheless an important example of the role of culture in the interplay of nation and
state. As Filewood very succinctly puts it:

> In Quebec the battle for sovereignty may have been lost in the ballot boxes, but it was won
> in the field of culture. Quebecois theatre research developed its project of exploring and
> theorising the layers of national history, thereby consolidating in its discourse borders
> that were much less secure in actuality.
>
> (Filewood 2004: 118)

In Filewood's analysis of theatre's role in the construction of a modern Quebecois identity we see an example of a recurrent claim in contemporary theatre scholarship, namely that theatre and performance become particularly important sights in the contestation of national identity when nationhood is not commensurate with statehood.

Of course, many would argue that the case of Quebec is not even the most significant site of struggle within the larger question of Canadian national identity, something with which Filewood himself implicitly agrees when he engages with what he sees as a fundamental failure of recent theatre history in Canada, asserting that '[i]t can be argued that the absence of First Nations theatre culture in Canadian theatre historiography has been a form of cultural genocide' (121).

Here is not the place to discuss the case of Canada in much detail, but there is a fundamental argument of central importance to this volume, namely that not only is theatre a potentially very potent force in opening up questions of identity in 'small' nations, but that such questions frequently need to go some way beyond the more obvious polarising questions of power relations in any given situation. This can at times open up areas that are less than comfortable and which are about the identity of small nations that have experienced versions of colonial oppression, but which nevertheless raise complex questions about the dominance of particular versions of new and emerging national identities.

What then can we hope to achieve by publishing a series of chapters on theatre and performance in small nations, as opposed simply to one on the relationship between theatre and nationalism in general? To begin with, the two things are intimately connected as we have already said, but there is strong case for arguing that small nations, particularly at a historical juncture in which a considerable number have 'emerged' or are emerging in various forms, have particular things to reveal about the relationship between culture and national identity.

Here it is worth emphasising the idea of small nationhood being defined at least partly by power relationships – particularly those that involve a colonial or quasi-colonial relationship to another state. This is what makes the case of Canada, geographically one of the largest nations on earth, so fascinating. Not only does the nation as a whole occupy a particular kind of position in relation to the United States, but Canada itself remains a member of the Commonwealth of Nations with the British monarch as its head of state. Furthermore, the province of Quebec raises issues on its own questions of nationhood intimately connected to questions of language while, as Filewood points out above, the engagement with ideas of First Nationhood is at an early stage of development.

The role of theatre in this kind of context is of potentially huge significance. In small nations the scope for meaningful proportions of the population to be involved with and affected by theatre's role in the construction of national identity is genuinely significant. Of course, this extends far beyond those that work in the theatre or actually attend performances. It includes the ways in which debates are conducted through forms of media, the ways in which culture is handled in political discourse and, of course, the ways in which theatre interacts with other cultural forms.

The contributors to this book will of course implicitly examine these claims in the radically different cultural contexts about which they write. For now though, it is important to explore some of the fundamental principles behind the relationship between theatre, performance and the identity of small nations as well as exploring further the usefulness and legitimacy of the category of 'small nations' itself.

In her examination of the 'performance' of national identity in the United Kingdom Jen Harvie reiterates clearly and usefully the key relationship between theatre, performance and national identity: 'A founding principle here is that national identities are neither biologically nor territorially given: rather they are creatively produced or staged' (Harvie 2005: 2). The metaphoric language is of course carefully chosen for its relationship to performance and Harvie goes on to make clear links to the work of both Benedict Anderson and the idea of the 'imagined community' (Anderson 1983) and Michael Billig whose idea of 'banal nationalism' usefully connects formal performance with the performative nature of 'everyday life' (Billig 1995).

For Billig, of course, Anderson's 'imagined community' is brought into being through the 'banal' performances of everyday life – eating, wearing clothes, watching sport and so on. In turn, as Harvie points out, this is what gives national identity its 'dynamic' quality (2005: 3). If people are constantly in the act of creating their identity then the 'nation' ceases to be a given monolithic entity and becomes instead a contested site, one that is potentially open to constant change and re-invention.

In the case of small nations, particularly those that have newly emerged, often from colonial or quasi-colonial existences, this sense of constant re-invention is perhaps of particular interest and likely to be more transparent and dynamic than in larger, more stable contexts. Perhaps, most importantly, the sense of empowerment that comes from the idea of national identity being 'imagined' and contested is likely to be closer to a felt reality in the context of small nations where the gap between those who create the nation in this fluid, everyday performative sense and those who enact the idea of the nation through its legislation and formal structures of power is likely to be so much smaller.

Bjorn Olaffson suggests that 'the citizen of a small state has a better possibility to influence decision making than a citizen in a large state' (Olaffson 1998: 14). While there is an obvious danger of over simplification in such a point, the advantage of the idea is that it places emphasis on the advantages of small nations, something that has been vital to the surge in interest in the idea of states that offer alternative models to the received wisdoms of globalisation and the hegemony of the superpower. As Hjort and Petrie put it:

An important feature of the literature on small nations, and particularly of those writings produced by members of small nations, is to call attention not only to the challenges of small nationhood, but also, potentially, to the opportunities [...] Small nationhood need not be a liability nor a clear sign of sub-optimality [...]

(Hjort and Petrie 2007: 7)

While a number of the contributors to this volume do indeed draw attention to the problems of small nationhood, particularly when the concept becomes entwined with the idea of the First Nation, there is also, in Europe at least, a sense that the contemporary theatrical culture of emergent small nations is of particular interest and indeed capable of a powerful questioning of received models and structures. This is particularly evident in the chapters on the stateless nations of Scotland and Wales.

A key justification for this volume, then, is that while theatre and performance are key objects of the study of national identity within all states, they are of particular interest in small nations. The proximity of the citizen (and therefore the artist) to the decision-making process in the way that Olaffson describes above is one key reason.

A second, already mentioned, but which now can be explored a little further is the idea that national identity within small nations has a tendency to be the subject of continual debate and contestation. This, when added to the enhanced significance of specifically cultural practices in nations that are often 'stateless' make the role of theatre and performance in the construction of small nations of particular interest.

During the period when Wales was debating the setting up of a national theatre in the English language the term 'national conversation' was one frequently used by the advocates of the use of public funding to assist in the process. Users of the term implied that a national theatre in the English language (Theatr Genedlaethol Cymru, operating in Welsh, was founded in 2003) was a potentially vital contributor to any conversation understood as part of the ongoing project of national understanding in a country that conducted its official business in two languages. The case of Wales is dealt with in one of the chapters that make up this volume, but this idea of theatre and performance as significant contributors to 'national conversations', particularly in small nations with complex relationships to larger, more powerful neighbours will now be examined a little further through a brief discussion of examples that are not covered elsewhere.

Of particular interest at the time of writing is an experiment in Denmark that describes itself as the 'Temporary National Theatre'. The organisation, according to its website:

> is an investigation into the nature and identity of 'national' theatre organised by directors *Anders Paulin, Mia Lipschitz* and architect *Tor Lindstrand* for the *Royal Danish Theatre* between 17 of October 2009–24 of April, 2010. The main objective of TNT is to examine multiple potentials for a cultural arena; understood as a public space where citizens and institution meet to define collective ideas of ethics, identity and social imagination. The program is being developed in co-operation with institutions and individuals from a diverse number of fields and disciplines. The more different perspectives, expertise, experiences and strategies that occupy a public space, the more impossible it gets for one identity to claim sovereignty as a dominant narrative. Thereby allowing for a temporary transformation of the national stage into a temporary house of the people.

> (http://www.temporarynationaltheatre.dk/)

Here we see some of the key contemporary ideas that surround progressive notions of national identity being enacted in the context of an 'official' experiment. Theatre and performance are being used as key elements in an open, democratic invitation to take part in a national conversation that is in itself the central defining metaphor for national identity. While 'Temporary National Theater' is by definition a short-lived experiment its aim is to leave a legacy of questioning and creative disruption of monolithic ideas about both the purpose of national theatres and national identity itself. One particular event in the six-month long experiment presented a particular challenge within the contemporary Western European context:

IT'S ALL NATIONAL has been organised as a series of events that will make the theatre available for conversations, presentations and entertainment as part of an inquiry into asylum policies in Denmark. A selection of guest artists, researchers, philosophers, lawyers, politicians and asylum seekers will be invited to present perspectives on stage with a wide range of positions and opinions about asylum policies and integration in Denmark. The aim is to provide a stage for asylum seekers and Danes for dialog, recognition, and understanding.

(http://www.temporarynationaltheatre.dk/)

Denmark's position as a 'small nation' is particularly interesting here. Writing about Danish film culture, Mette Hjort says, 'If lack of confidence is a typical marker of small nationhood, then Denmark would appear to have transcended its small-nation status in recent years [...]' (Hjort 2007: 25). While the idea of 'lack of confidence' as a defining characteristic is a tempting one with a lot to recommend it, it is perhaps worth speculating for a moment on a modification to the idea. 'Lack of confidence' tends to suggest a negative, a hesitancy that hampers progress in the macho world of international politics (and culture). However, if the idea changes to one of a lack of 'certainty' and extends to a willingness to question and debate, then Denmark's example (along with others) takes on a different meaning.

The Crucible, Arthur Miller's great allegory of resistance to state-sponsored 'certainty' has frequently been associated with the lines from W. B. Yeats' *The Second Coming* (see, for example, Welland 1979: 57):

The best lack all conviction, while the worst/are full of a passionate intensity

The 'anti-certainty' of the Danish Temporary National Theatre experiment is a clear example of the role of theatre in the construction of small nationhood that seeks not to define, but to invite debate and to empower, particularly among those for whom conventional notions of national identity are a potential difficulty.

In an article specifically devoted to the idea of 'staging the nation', Zoltan Imre spells out what he sees as an essential problem in a globalised world:

[...]one of the main challenges facing the European nation-states and their institutions today, especially within the borders of the European Union, is how to present the various discourses, views, and perspectives of their diverse communities on national and international levels.

(Imre 2008: 85)

The example of the Danish National Theatre in hosting its 'temporary' version is one imaginative response to such a challenge, albeit temporary and transient. As Imre suggests, emergent European nations, some of which are discussed in the chapters that follow, are attempting to use public funding as an instrument to create new models of national theatres that exist as constant reminders of the challenges of contemporary national identity. Such models, he suggests, despite theatre's relative marginality in contemporary culture, have the potential to open up the kinds of spaces within which people can rediscover an appetite for democratic engagement with ideas that shape our imagined communities and identities. After discussing the National Theatre of Scotland as one such model, Imre states:

What this fragmentary view of a national theatre tends to suggest is that even in today's post-industrial, post-socialist, and globalised world, when theatre in general is a marginal commodity in a capitalist cultural industry, *national theatre* projects can still draw people, parties, groups, and institutions as participants in debates, demonstrations, and panels on what it might be or should be within their real or virtual walls. As a result, the current advocates of national theatre projects might be able to transform an old idea and an old institution into new methodological territories and alternative sites where the status quo can be reconsidered, and where the constant (re) constructions of nationhood, nationality, and national identity can be analyzed and understood. We shall see [...]

(Imre 2008: 89)

The conception of this volume, then, rests, at least partly, on the idea that it is within small nations and first nations that some of the most interesting work is taking place inside of the very broad arena of using theatre and performance as a sophisticated means of scrutinising questions of nationhood, nationalism and national identity in the age of globalisation.

Though Imre's words above are concerned most specifically with variations on national theatre institutions, this book offers ways in which a similar role to the one he suggests for theatre and performance can be found in different contexts, but in a wider sense than 'national theatres' implies. While 'national theatres' are important, as many of the contributors suggest, there are also many other ways in which theatre and performance are offering challenging new ways to consider ideas of the nation and its role in the formation of the identities of its citizens.

What follows attempts to explain the very difficult process of selection that went into assembling a collection that could never be genuinely representative of the huge variety of contexts in which the kinds of debates that are outlined above exist. This said, there were real efforts made to assemble a variety of not only political or geographical contexts, but of approaches to the whole question of nationhood and the final section of this introduction tries to provide insight into at least some of the questions that such a process inevitably begs.

What then could the brief to contributors of this volume realistically be? Perhaps more important still, how does one go about soliciting contributions when the idea of the small nation is a contested one and definable in a number of ways?

One answer is that this volume is one that hopes to articulate questions about the boundaries of the idea of small nationhood and therefore of the relationship of small nations to their theatrical culture. In order to do this, the contributors take a wide range of approaches, both in terms of the contexts from which they write and the dimension of theatre and performance that they seek to address.

If the idea of the nation itself is a contested one, then the term 'small nation' takes the problem a stage further. Moreover, in a volume that includes work on a nation as geographically enormous as Australia and as populous as Malaysia, some further discussion is necessary at this point.

To begin with it is vital to repeat that no single all-encompassing definition of the 'small nation' is being attempted. Rather this is a collection that offers key case studies of different approaches to the idea of small nationhood specifically in relation to aspects of the theatre and performance work that takes place in such very different settings. As has already been stated, if there is a single dominant factor it is the question of power and the nation's recent history with regard to questions of subjugation and division, frequently in colonial or quasi-colonial settings.

As the very idea of small nationhood has taken at least a fragile hold in international scholarship there have of course been attempts at definitions, though very few, within the disciplines of Theatre and Performance. To some extent this reflects the fact that the idea of the 'national' has been perhaps rather less significant in the history of Theatre and Performance scholarship than it has in, say, Film Studies, where work on 'national cinemas' has been central. This is of course not to deny the importance of 'the nation' within the broad scope of theatre historiography and, in particular, there has been significant recent work on the emergence and significance of the idea of the national theatre such as Wilmer (2008) and Jones (2007).

Even within Film Studies though, where the sub-discipline of 'national cinema' is so well-established, there has been, until very recently, little work on the idea of the small nation and cinema. In Mette Hjort and Duncan Petrie's pioneering work on cinema and small nations they state that:

[...] for the most part the concept of small nation has not been central to the concerns of film scholars, who have yet to engage with the rich literature on the topic produced by other disciplines. Small nationhood figures mostly as a general intuition, rather than a clearly defined analytic tool, in the work of film scholars.

(2007: 3)

Interestingly though, one of the examples of intuitive engagement with the idea of small nationhood that Hjort and Petrie explore, is strongly illustrative of the problematic involved in the concept for all disciplines. Referring the reader to Bordwell and Thompson's classic text (2003: 3) they observe that '[c]ountries referred to in this short section on "Smaller Producing Countries" include Mexico, India, Colombia, New Zealand, Australia, Ireland and Canada'.

As Hjort and Petrie observe, such a collection is arrived at by equating the idea of 'small' levels of cinematic production with any definition of small nationhood and even in this respect it would have to refer to India only within a very limited historical time-frame. This, however, is not to deny the insight that such a perspective may offer and, though its definition of small nation is not as broad as Bordwell and Thompson's, this book clearly presents chapters that are a challenge to many existing conceptions of the idea of 'small'.

Usefully, Hjort and Petrie go on to rehearse the case for a number of potential objective measures of small nationhood – population size, geographical scale, gross national product and, most interestingly the concept of power relations from the work of Miroslav Hroch:

> We only designate as small nations those which were in subjection to a ruling nation for such a long period that the relation of subjection took on a structural character for both parties.
>
> (Hroch 1985: 9)

Hjort and Petrie then attempt to construct a selection of 'case studies' based upon the four criteria above without, in a sense, attempting to delineate any kind of hierarchy of importance. The effect of this is to introduce the idea of objective criteria while never quite owning up to the impossibility of such a thing. Indeed Hjort and Petrie claim that '*The Cinema of Small Nations* presents a multifaceted working definition of small nationhood encompassing four indicators of size' (Hjort and Petrie 2007: 6).

This is very useful, but tends to gloss over the fact that such 'facets' can sometimes be directly contradictory with, for example, Iceland's population and geographical scale being miniscule, but with a GNP that is much higher than many countries with far larger areas and populations. Far better perhaps to present the contradictions for what they are and, most importantly for what they can teach us about the idea of nationhood and, in this context, about the relationship of theatre and performance to questions of identity in such contexts.

Here then, while taking note of the criteria proposed by Hjort and Petrie, the chapters offer a number of radically different approaches to the idea of 'small' nation with only the proviso that they shed different light on the question to that provided by the other contributors. In many cases this comes simply from the inherent differences between the national case studies that make up the volume, and this will be discussed below. In others however, there is a more radical questioning of the idea of nationhood and an engagement with the strong emergence of the idea of First Nations.

For some scholars of First Nationhood, a simple equation with the idea of small nations would be highly problematic and that is not what is intended in this volume. However to ignore the obvious potential for rich dialogue between the two ideas would have been a greater omission. It is therefore around the common ground of relationships to centres of large national powers (mainly through the legacy of colonialism) that chapters that deal with First and small nations are here presented alongside each other in the spirit of a search for the multifaceted significance of theatre and performance in certain kinds of national contexts.

In 2009 London held its first festival of 'First Nations creative arts'. Its website opens with a quotation from a nineteenth-century leader of the Metis people, by then a part of the administrative territory of Canada: "'My people will sleep for one hundred years, when they awake it will be the artists who give them their spirit back" Louis Riel (Metis leader, Canada, 1885)' (http://www.originsfestival.bordercrossings.org.uk/Default.aspx). As well as asserting the centrality of art forms in the struggle for the survival of First Nations, the website goes on to position the festival not as folk-art curiosity but rather part of an effort to use art forms and subsequent opportunities for dialogue as a means of foregrounding the potential of small and First nations to provide examples to a wider world besieged it seems by the threat of environmental disaster and violent conflict:

At a time when the Western world faces environmental and financial crisis, can it learn from the respectful relationships the indigenous peoples of the world have with the Earth, within their own communities and with their heritage? Origins invites audiences and performers to engage in this dialogue in London, capital of a country that radically changed history for the original inhabitants of the lands it 'discovered' and colonised in centuries past.

(http://www.originsfestival.bordercrossings.org.uk/Default.aspx)

In some ways this rationale for 'Origins: Festival of First Nations' has a strong relationship with the rationale for this volume and the series of which it is part. The range of contexts that are covered in the individual chapters necessarily means that not all small nations aspire to the same sense of 'difference' asserted above. However, there are fundamental ways in which the media and culture of small nations (and First Nations) ask questions about a globalised world in which difference is often felt to be erased and, through an examination of aspects of theatre and performance practices, the contributors to this volume seek to shed light on those questions.

There is no question that the volume is somewhat skewed towards the United Kingdom and Ireland. In certain respects this is entirely intentional. This book originated in the Centre for the Study of Media and Culture in Small Nations based at the University of Glamorgan in Cardiff, South Wales. The Centre's principal aim was to use research experience of one context, Wales, to create dialogue between small nations that would shed light on what could be learned from the collective experience of such contexts.

The creation of a Wales Assembly Government in 1999 following the referendum on devolved powers in 1997 (and the parallel, though different processes of devolution to the

Scottish Parliament and Northern Ireland Assembly) has clearly provided a clearer overall context for debates about Wales's status as a nation, and in turn raised interest in the way that the country can be compared to other contexts within Europe, such as Catalonia or Galicia in Spain.

In Wales and Scotland, in particular, this process of political devolution has resulted in the creation of new national institutions for theatre and performance as well as the very direct involvement of artists in the profound questions around the representation of national identity that such events inevitably raise. The somewhat ironically titled 'United Kingdom' does then present an opportunity to examine newly created small national contexts that are in close proximity and therefore constant dialogue with one another. This is especially true in the case of the National Theatre of Scotland and National Theatre Wales, both of which have adopted radical non-building-based models that they hope reflect the kind of democratic engagement that is in the spirit of their newly devolved nations.

In the case of the United Kingdom's close neighbour (and former colony), Ireland, questions of identity and the small nation are considered not in the context of the renewed confidence that devolved powers brought to Scotland and Wales, but rather in the midst of what a worldwide recession has brought to a country that had become a symbol of what a small nation might achieve economically and culturally. The phrase 'Celtic Tiger' has so quickly metamorphosed from a badge of pride (in some quarters at least) to a hollow symbol of the false dawn of economic growth that has left behind so many casualties. Cathy Leeney's chapter then is less an affirmation of the imagined Irish community and more a questioning of the idea of nation. At the end of her chapter she asks: 'Can the theatre of a small nation maintain its value if the small nation effectively no longer exists?'

In the case of the other European contexts represented here, there are also striking contrasts that are, to say the least, sobering. Helena Buffery's account of the contemporary Catalan stage both recognises the confidence of the strong contemporary theatre scene and at the same time explores the potential conflict between a quest for connection with the 'universal' in art and the desire to maintain the integrity of the 'local', in this case small nation identity. The choice to do this partly through an examination of contemporary productions of the play *Hamlet*, that is most frequently touted as the touchstone of universality in world literature, is bold and one that yields powerful insights into the potential for translation, as she puts it, to become

[…] a zone of intercultural encounter in which meaning is negotiated between source and target languages, providing a two-way mirror in which to glimpse the cultural order and resistance of the source culture, too.

Here we see not only an examination of a small stateless nation, but also the dynamics of cultural power as Catalan productions cast light on the potentially hegemonic power of the idea of Shakespeare as universal.

Australia and New Zealand, so often carelessly paired in discussions about everything from global economics to international sport, are here presented as contrasting studies of the relationship between theatre, performance and some of the multiple identities that make up these complex postcolonial societies. For Sharon Mazer, writing in New Zealand, it appears that, '[i]n this small nation we seem sometimes to be perpetually remaking ourselves into ever smaller mini-nations-within-the-nation'. As she goes on to say, this is perhaps the inevitable outcome of the kind of colonial history that both Australia and New Zealand possess and the consequent contemporary dialogue over forms of material and symbolic reparation.

As well as providing a series of thorough insights into the evolution of theatre as a response to evolving ideas of New Zealand nationhood, Mazer is usefully very explicit about the unique specific contribution that theatre and performance can make to debates about small nationhood (as opposed to more general questions about the contribution of all art forms):

[…] one of the first stages in the journey from colony to country – if not the establishment of a national theatre – seems to be the theatricalisation of a national identity. For Gilbert and Tompkins: 'The multiply-coded representational systems of theatre offer a variety of opportunities for the recuperation of a post-colonial subjectivity which is not simply inscribed in written discourse but embodied through performance.'

There are notes of caution, too. Writing in Wales where the discourse of rugby union is commonplace, Mazer's invocation of the traditional Maori 'war dance' performed before all New Zealand All Black rugby games carries a special force:

Like the haka, Maori theatre seems to have come to dominate the international imagination about New Zealand's national identity, albeit in ways that are perhaps less about empowerment than about branding.

New Zealand is alone in this volume of course in opening up questions both about a postcolonial small nation and its 'internal' Maori first nation. Mazer's chapter is therefore both highly complex and very valuable in opening up the multi-layered complexities of national identity in New Zealand that offer valuable insights that resonate across all postcolonial societies.

Rea Dennis also writes about a nation with questions of first nationhood at the forefront of any discussion of its overall national identity. Australia as a whole however has an entirely different relationship to the idea of small nationhood as Dennis makes clear near the start of her chapter:

Since September 11, Australia's engagement in the war on terror has led to a visceral exploitation of fragments of identity narrative. This has come in many forms, yet at its most basic appears as a question about the balance between the pursuit of our national security and the sanctity of our human rights.

Alongside Australia's postcolonial status and national acts of reparation such as Sorry Day and Reconciliation week, one has to consider the nation's membership of the Anglo-American dominated Western group of nations and all that this implies. As Dennis revealingly recounts, while the spectacular 'performance' of Australian national identity at the 2000 Sydney Olympics suggested a country moving towards peace with itself and its relationship with its first nation population, subsequent events, especially post-9/11 point to much more complex unresolved narratives. Using the case studies of two performances centrally concerned with both personal and national identities, Dennis opens up those narratives and offers a complex picture of a culture tested by the polarities of international recognition and unresolved internal conflicts over national identity.

Teresa Marrero's essay about Latin@/Hispanic theatre in the United States not only provides the volume with a radically different context for the discussion of small and First nationhood, it also offers a pertinent reminder of the role of academic writing in the construction (and sometimes constriction) of communities:

Because scholarship contributes to the production of collective identities (or lack thereof), as such, imagined academic communities establish spheres of intellectual influence that, in turn, bestow value upon the production of certain nations versus others, thus influencing not only self perception but that of others.

Within the unimaginably complex context of the relationship between the United States and all its constituent communities, scholarship of this kind necessitates an even more nuanced sensitivity to the history and politics of national formations than is usually the case. Marrero's essay admirably displays such sensitivity, while also leaving us in little doubt of the almost intractable complexity of discussing such matters to the satisfaction of all communities and the artists that work within them.

Perhaps of all the contributions to this volume it is Teresa Marrero's essay that (at least implicitly) asks the most difficult question about the limits of the construct 'small nation'. Writing from within the largest state of one of the most powerful nations on earth, Marrero's case study is a less than obvious comparator to Wales or even New Zealand to take just two examples. However, by discussing some of the same fundamental questions about the way that artists frame questions of power, the role of language and their relationship to audiences with competing ideas about national identity, the chapter helps to place the debates that the volume hopes to ignite within a new framework. There is no doubt that to some the idea of small nation carries clear connotations of the quaint or quirky, with traditional folk art to the fore. The discussion of competing national identities in places such as Dallas is an important corrective.

The most clear and explicit connection between racial and national identities is made by Susan Mary Philips's chapter on English-language theatre in Malaysia. Philips of course begins by questioning strongly the ways in which the idea of race has been used and constructed, particularly as part of the colonial experience, but also acknowledges its continuing contemporary relevance to Malaysian politics and culture, even as its usefulness or legitimacy as a way of thinking about populations comes under increasing scrutiny.

For Philips the enduring Malaysian preoccupation with restrictive racial constructs remains a problem and one, for her, that introduces a negative connotation to the idea of Malaysia as a small nation:

> In terms of size, population and economy, Malaysia is unquestionably a small nation. However, I would argue that it is also a small nation in terms of how it deals with issues of race. Situated in a geographical location which has led to its constantly being exposed to a myriad cultural and racial influences, it yet seeks to retreat within narrow and limiting racial and cultural boundaries, thus imposing a kind of involuntary smallness and narrowness on its inhabitants.

In this context then Philips sees theatre makers as key dissenting voices, capable of unsettling an outmoded way of thinking that, in her words 'has taken deep root in the Malaysian psyche'. In many ways the least optimistic of the chapters, certainly in terms of the impact of artist's voices on progressive understanding of a small nation's identity, nevertheless Philips does identify examples of theatre that resist the essentialism that she identifies as being at the heart of the 'official' Malay construction of national identity.

Finally, in a chapter on probably the least well-known national context in the volume, Aparna Sharma considers the case of Assam in North-east India as an example of what she calls 'micro-nationalism', a phenomenon that has been part of the national picture in India since the end of British colonial rule in 1947. Sharma's approach is distinct from most of the other chapters in its concentration on one form of ritual performance, the *Bihu* dance, as a prism through which to see the complex picture of Assam nationalism, one that attempts to interrogate more widely circulated representations of the nationalist phenomena which are often refracted through militarist discourses.

For Sharma one of the key problems of the micro-nationalist movement in India is the lack of both resources and commitment on the part of the mainstream Indian media to encourage the understanding of nationalist aspirations. This is particularly true of a region such as Assam that is geographically and culturally remote from the main Indian centres of population and political power. Sharma's focus on the *Bihu* dance specifically and the *Bohag-Bihu* spring time festival in Assam more generally is designed to reveal how performance is one of the key ways in which more fluid and progressive notions of micro-nationalism are enacted. As the dance and the festival have adapted to new urban contexts they have carried with them the continuity to past traditions and have therefore become central to contemporary ideas of Assamese national identity:

> No longer primarily ritualistic in terms of agricultural links, *Bohag Bihu* festivities are entwined with the dynamics of cultural identity formation within the micro-nationalist

context of Assam, serving to symbolise and evoke Assamese folk culture as a way to define and assert Assamese identity within the wider rubric of modern nationhood.

As India's power and influence in the world community as one of the so-called 'BRIC' countries (Brazil, Russia, India and China) increases, the collective memory of its former colonised status recedes somewhat. Aparna Sharma's chapter is a timely reminder that the complexities of the colonial era now leave behind other forms of nationalist aspiration for Indian politicians to negotiate. For artists in turn this frequently involves fascinating dialogue between contemporary international influence and the multi-layered traditions embedded in micro-nationalist contexts.

Slightly different in tone from the other more traditional chapters of academic analysis, Goran Stefanovski's account of a writer's negotiation of the effective disintegration of national cultures over two decades in the Balkans is an often very moving account of struggle to survive at all, both personally and in terms of any idea of a national theatre and performance culture. Stefanovski's account is a highly personal essay focusing on what he calls the 'ex-Yugoslavia', but to some extent reflecting on the whole of an Eastern Europe that has created large numbers of 'new' nations in the last 20 years.

Stefanovski's writer's perspective is invigorating and occasionally startling. It is brutally honest, not just about the conflict that caused his own migration and crisis of identity, but also about the reaction of the west:

When I first arrived in England, as Sarajevo was burning, I met a well-meaning producer who wanted to cash in on my story and made no secret about it. She told me: 'Goran, you're an asset now. But it'll only last six months. You must hurry up.'

In Stefanovski's analysis the situation in the Balkans (and in so much of Eastern Europe) remains so fluid that all he is able to do is offer an often poetic meditation on what the crisis has felt like for an established theatre maker who has had their world torn apart:

Eastern Europe is desperately trying to reinvent itself and define its new identity. Its artists are waking up from a historical narcosis. They are rubbing their eyes, shaking off their delusions and resetting their memory. They are looking at the clock to check the time, feeling around to check the place. They are gazing at themselves in the mirror, bewildered. They wonder what to wear: 'What do I want to look like? Who am I?'

Stefanovski's account is not so concerned with detached analysis, but its fluidity, its flashes of anger and its often very black humour seem to offer insights that make a valuable contribution to the breadth and variety of approach that characterise the collection.

As has already been indicated, the selection of nations for a volume of restricted length such as this one will inevitably leave some large gaps. However, there can never realistically be a promise of true global representation, particularly after a historical period when small nations have proliferated and in which rapidly changing global economics are causing very significant shifts in world economic and political power. There has been a real effort to balance on the one hand the volume's firm roots in the small nations of the United Kingdom and on the other a genuine desire to explore as wide a variety as possible of contrasting small and first nation situations.

In addition there has also been an effort made to include work that looks across a wide spectrum of theatre and performance. The volume is inevitably heavy with consideration of the national theatre institutions and the ways that some small nations have led the world in offering radically different ways in which such institutions can operate. It is a key way in which the progressive possibilities of small nationhood have become expressed. The volume also clearly demonstrates that national theatres are very definitely only one dimension to the vital role that theatre and performance plays in the continuing imagination of national identities. From the folk-rituals of Assam to Playback Theatre in Australia and the translation and adaptation of Shakespeare in Catalonia (and much more), the individual authors here offer what I see as a rich and varied selection of examinations of the vitality of the role of theatre and performance in the making and continuous remaking of small nations across the globe. It inevitably raises more questions than it can possibly answer, but if it makes an effective contribution to a fascinating emerging area of international scholarship, the effort will have been worth it.

Works cited

Anderson, B. (1983), *Imagined Communities: Reflections on the Origin and Spread of Nationalism*, London: Verso.

Billig, M. (1995), *Banal Nationalism*, London: Sage.

Border Crossings, http://www.originsfestival.bordercrossings.org.uk/Default.aspx. Accessed June 2010.

Bordwell, D., and K. Thompson (2003), *Film History: An Introduction*, London: McGraw-Hill.

Burcharth, M. (2006), 'Denmark's problem with Muslims', *New York Times*, 12 February, http://www.nytimes.com/2006/02/12/opinion/12iht-edoped.html. Accessed June 2010).

Filewood, A. (2004), 'Deregimenting Canadian Theatre History', in S. E. Wilmer (ed.), *Writing and Re-Writing National Theatre Histories*, Iowa City: University of Iowa Press, Chapter 7, pp. 106–126.

Gilbert, H. (2004), 'Foreward' to Lo, J. (2004), *Staging Nation: English Language Theatre in Malaysia and Singapore*, Hong Kong: Hong Kong University Press, p. vii.

Harvie, J. (2005), *Staging the UK*, Manchester: Manchester University Press.

Hjort, M. (2007), 'Denmark', in Hjort M. and Petrie D. (ed.), *The Cinema of Small Nations*, Edinburgh: Edinburgh University Press, pp. 23–42.

Hjort, M., and Petrie, D. (2007), *The Cinema of Small Nations*, Edinburgh: Edinburgh University Press.

Hroch, M. (1985), *The Social Preconditions of National Revival in Europe: A Comparative Analysis of the Social Composition of Patriotic Groups Among the Smaller European Nations*, Cambridge: Cambridge University Press.

Imre, Z. (2008), 'Staging the Nation: Changing Concepts of a National Theatre in Europe', *New Theatre Quarterly*, 24: 1 (February), pp. 75–94.

Jones, A. (2007), *National Theatres in Context: France, Germany, England and Wales*, Cardiff, University of Wales Press.

Olaffson, B. (1998), *Small States in the Global System: Analysis and Illustrations from the Case of Iceland*, Aldershot: Ashgate.

http://www.temporarynationaltheatre.dk/. Accessed June 2010.

Welland, D. (1979), *Miller The Playwright* (3rd edition), London: Methuen.

Wilmer, S. (2008), *National Theatres in a Changing Europe*, Basingstoke: Palgrave Macmillan.

Chapter 1

Location, Location, Location: Plays and Realities: Living Between the Pre-modern and the Postmodern in Irish Theatre

Cathy Leeney

This chapter is part of a broader argument about how Irish theatre and performance confronts the post-human condition in the twenty-first century, how it reflects upon and explores the experience of living after humanist values. Here, I try to deal with more specific issues of space and identity in plays written during and after the Celtic Tiger period in Ireland, the period of economic hyper-development that is often dated from the early 1990s to about 2008.

In Ireland it is commonly understood that the history of theatre has been closely associated with the assertion of national identity. Dion Boucicault, in the middle of the nineteenth century, created challenges to colonising English stereotypes of Irishness, while reassuring audiences that a *modus vivendi* was possible and desirable between landed and peasant classes and between the neighbouring islands. Later, theatres staged new visions of the myths and images of a self-consciously separate Irishness, and, even when playwrights had other issues on their minds, Irish audiences and critics stepped in with some consistency seeing identity everywhere as a defining theme. Conflicts resulting from the partition of the island of Ireland into the Republic's 26 counties and Northern Ireland's six counties have prolonged concerns with identity as they applied to the culture clash between Unionist and Nationalist interests and agendas; issues of identity turned inwards, were often defensive and focussed on exclusion.

Through the latter part of the twentieth century (and powerfully at play long before then) influences from the wider world have impacted on the experience of being Irish. Declan Hughes, who was born in the 1960s, is one of the first critics specifically to articulate the gap between official versions of Irish identity and the felt experience of growing up with Americanised or internationalised culture as the key reference point. Seeing that the pressure on national identity had already won the contest, his argument is that

[t]here are two ways of reacting to the perceived collapse of cultural identities [...] One is, literally, to react: to insist on national and regional identity authenticity [...] the second way of reacting [is] to reflect it, to embrace it, to see it as liberating. It's the condition.

(Hughes 1999: 11, 14)

Although Mary Manning and Tom Murphy, amongst others, had earlier dramatised Irish people's passionate and sometimes painful ties with other cultural contexts, Hughes expressed a generation's alienation from the national identity values promoted by state agencies, and he described a growing sense of disjunction between an ideological localism and an actual globalism. Aspirations towards the images of internationalism had, for Hughes and his peers, replaced the hegemonic prescriptions of church and state, which in Ireland's case were deeply and damagingly integrated. There is nothing unusual about this development, as most small nations feel the pressure of new colonising forces, and probably nothing unusual about its effect on Irish playwriting and theatre making. From a conservatively nationalist Irish point of view, the colonising pressures of England had merely been replaced by those of international capital and multinational enterprise. But is some more radical and complex change taking place that goes further than another kind of colonisation from another source? Is Irish theatre, sometimes tacitly sometimes explicitly, enquiring into human identity as it grows out of rootedness, place, history and community by exploring how it is uprooted, displaced, adrift in the present moment and amidst new definitions of place and community?

The difficulty of totalising analysis in this postmodern context is obvious. It is not possible to reflect the range of kinds of theatre being made in Ireland, to include a properly representative range of plays, dance theatre, devised performance, outdoor spectacle and live art. The material here makes reference to the work of a limited selection of playwrights whose plays bear relation to the idea that identity has migrated from the idea of nation to become a shared concern circling the issue of place and its role in contextualising identity and connecting individuals into communities.

The writer, journalist and theatre critic Fintan O'Toole has argued convincingly that in the twentieth century, Ireland jumped from being pre-modern (or pre-industrial) to being postmodern/post-industrial, missing out on the intermediary stage (O'Toole 2003). He is describing how, in Ireland, the unselfconsciously traditional might be found cheek by jowl with the latest high technology systems and communications. The phenomenon is not unique to Ireland and has been noted across the developing world. In the 1970s an English author told me that his visit to Dublin felt to him like travelling to any regional English city trapped in a time warp in the 1950s. To him Ireland merely lagged behind. But since then time has become far more fractured. During the Celtic Tiger period of economic boom, the Irish may have begun to believe their own publicity – that not only did Ireland offer an unparalleled quality of life and unrivalled opportunities for enjoyment and 'craic', but that they could also wield economic power matching the audacity, greed and high earnings of any other national élite. Those who won success at that time might move with ease between the pre-modern world of their grandparents, perhaps materially poor but supposedly rich in cultural and spiritual resources, and the postmodern sophistication of highly technologised communication, travel and international business and property interests. This sense of movement, this 'between-ness', has, I will argue, become a key image in Irish theatre. Its impact on the setting and structure of plays places new emphasis on a new enquiry: What is it to be one of those who can shrug off one world to enter another, without any burden of commitment, history or vulnerability? There is also a new question: Who are we without a sense of place and how does theatre deal with this?

In what follows I wish to explore location in the dramatic space of plays, by which I mean the location and spatial contexts of the play as indicated in the text, but not as interpreted by a scenographer in a specific production. My argument relies on recognising how spatial organisation lies at the heart of the semiotics of performance, that spatial context definitively frames the engagement of the audience with narrative, character and the process of making meaning on stage. From Artaud to Copeau to Brook, space defines theatre and the act of performance, while the theatre semiotician Anne Ubersfeld famously equates theatre with space. Defending the analysis of the dramatic space of a play on the basis of the text alone, Gay McAuley argues that '[a] great deal of information about spatial function is contained in the written playtext, and [...] reveal[s] the importance of the category of space in theatrical meaning making' (1999: 9). A central part of my concern is the relationship between dramatic space and place, that is to say, as Ciáran Benson defines it, 'what human beings make of space and time'. The process whereby persons develop identity through their bodily and shared connections with space, 'the subjectification of space and time' (2001: 7), Benson argues, is key to the formation of self. He quotes E. S. Casey:

Where we are – the place we occupy, [...] has everything to do with what and who we are (and finally that we are).

(1993: xiii)

Yet, it seems evident that many Irish playwrights are no longer in the business of representing place as key to the workings of their plays, the rooting of character and the contextualising of narrative. How then do they express this field of uncertainty, where space takes over from place? How do they create opportunities for performance to embody, for audiences, the unstable relationship between space, place and identity?

If audiences live in a state of between-ness: between history and virtuality, identity and performativity, narrative and intertextuality, spontaneous action and self-conscious reflexivity, hierarchised structure and postmodern playfulness, between the pre-modern and the postmodern, how does contemporary theatre explore their quandary? Does the term 'liminality' suffice any longer to express the unresolved state of the human subject, detached, freed and exhilarated perhaps, loosed into non-place? The contemporary Irish playwrights here wrote in the shadow of their predecessors, for example, J. M. Synge, Sean O'Casey and John B. Keane, who exploited dramatic space to dramatise specific lives as lived in specific locations, linking, often in complex ways, the places with the lives and exploring how they are entwined. The representation of what were once unfamiliar, authentic places on stage however has become a problem. As Garry Hynes points out in relation to staging John B. Keane's plays, '[i]f you go for some kind of realism you're suddenly part of the heritage industry' (2001: 200). The imagery of Keane's rural way of life has been co-opted into the marketing of brand Ireland and can no longer be seen outside that frame.

Brian Friel's Ballybeg, the location of several of his dramas, is at once a locale and an archetypal community. Friel reveals the restrictions and the (mostly lost) potentials of such social formations, their disequilibrium, and the grip kept on individuals' dreams. Yet, building on his abiding fascination with fluid stage space, in *Faith Healer* (1979) Friel achieves a very different kind of dramatic space. Here, locales proliferate and become confused; their names are an incantation, an emotional contour rather than a geographical one, and crucially the play is acted out in an imagined space of performance. The key moments of the narrative are located in highly specific detail though; in this sense, place eventually catches up with Frank Hardy when his fate materialises with utter inevitability, outside Ballybeg:

> [t]he yard was a perfect square enclosed by the back of the building and three high walls. [...] In the corners facing me and within the walls were two mature birch trees and the wind was sufficient to move them.
>
> (Friel 1984: 375)

The uncertainties surrounding location as the audience try to piece together Frank's, Grace's and Teddy's versions of events give rise to questions of character, narrative and truth that mark the play as reflexively postmodern. As Declan Kiberd observes, '[t]he play turns out to be about itself' (1996: 631). The space of the play is the space of performance, and for the three figures on stage, each isolated in a pool of light, it is a kind of limbo. *Faith Healer* draws attention to a dramaturgical strategy that unfixes the figure from the context: direct address to the audience. The argument is sometimes made that the popularity of monologue performance has economic motives, but might playwrights choose the single speaking figure to express detachment from place and its contextualising power? Perhaps the solo performer signals the era of non-place and its contest with place? The metatheatrical impact of monologue places the audience as silent and self-conscious interlocutors, while it also reflects contemporary experiences of the irresolution of space into place through mobile phones and other digital communications.

Several of the playwrights discussed in this chapter require particular settings for their dramas, and yet build in a sense of unease with fixed and steadfast place. They achieve this in a variety of ways. Dramaturgically speaking, space and time are always closely relative: inconstancy in temporal reference has the power to disrupt the coherence of dramatic space. Contextualising settings may be interrupted by sounds from elsewhere, by darkness, or by illogical or incoherent elements that break the frame, creating gaps that destabilise. Settings may combine realist and expressionist elements in an ill-fitting jigsaw of signs, or may present a hyper-realist image where each individual object points towards its narrative use.

The general principle of uncertainty in space, time and narrative has been brought to a new level in the Irish theatre of Martin McDonagh. His hybrid Irish/English identity (he grew up in London with Irish emigrant parents and spent holidays in Sligo and Connemara) unsettles distinctions between Irishness and Englishness, and as Fintan O'Toole observes, McDonagh is 'part of a generation that has completely redefined the term "Anglo-Irish" [... as] a new kind of fusion that arises, not from ascendency but from exile' (O'Toole, 1999: ix–x). McDonagh's drama first hit Irish stages in 1996 and swiftly became a phenomenon in Ireland

and England before *The Beauty Queen of Leenane* won four Tony awards on Broadway. It is not too much to say that Garry Hynes' Druid Theatre Company productions have become legendary in recent Irish theatre history as a defining marker of the process of globalisation (Lonergan 2009: 101–127).

From 1996 to 2001 McDonagh's plays had in common their west of Ireland settings, their use of Hiberno-English sentence structures and a series of intertextual references to Irish and other dramatic literatures. In 2003, *The Pillowman* was directed by John Crowley at the National Theatre (London), although McDonagh dates the play to 1994, prior to the staging of his other work; and a draft of the play was read at Druid's theatre space in Galway in 1997 (Lonergan 2009: 102). One way or another, *The Pillowman*, while it is significantly different in style and tone, contains dramaturgical strategies at their fullest development, strategies that are also present, in less developed form, in the work of the west of Ireland. Thus, the earlier-produced plays are usefully re-read through the later one.

The Pillowman operates in the interstices between show and tell, in theatre terms, between performance and narrative. Katurian is an abattoir worker and part-time story writer who is being interrogated by two policemen. Parts of the opening dialogue pastiche the clichés of television crime drama, but the scene quickly moves into a more threatening mood, echoing Pinter's *One for the Road*. From the moment when the '*[s]ound of a man screaming hideously a few rooms away*'[1] (McDonagh 2003: 23) breaks the action on the stage, the relationship between what is heard or told and what is seen or enacted becomes more and more deeply unreliable and disturbing. A kind of contest is set up between the value of the story and the sacrificial value of human suffering. Finally, McDonagh twists the ending to play out a retrospective victory of story over sacrifice when Katurian's brain-damaged brother, Michal, says he would prefer to live and suffer his parents' torture rather than lose Katurian's stories, which were inspired by Michal's pain. Leaving aside the moral implications of the play, the space of performance operates in a bizarre way. It shifts between recognisable accessories such as police files and institutional furniture, and is taken over by Katurian as he tells the story of his parents' experiment, and enacts his own words assisted by them. In Act I, Scene 2, Katurian sits '*in an approximation of a child's room*' (31); he narrates two versions of his parents' behaviour, which are acted out as he speaks. He presents the first version titled 'The Writer and the Writer's Brother' as if it were one of his stories. In the second version, 'The Truer Story' (34), Katurian finds his brother alive but physically and mentally damaged, and smothers his parents. Again, at the end of Act II, Scene 1, Katurian's story leads to him suffocating his brother, and Scene 2 comprises the story of the foster-parents and the girl who is Jesus; he '*narrates the story that the girl and the parents act out*' (67). Act III begins with Katurian's confession and death, but both dead brothers are resurrected to tell the final story of Michal's choice. Story and the demands of narrative shape enactment; the play questions the playwright's power – not only to write a story but also to shape an enactment. In *The Pillowman*, Katurian's key role as victim and as protagonist/dramaturg makes explicit McDonagh's fascinated self-awareness as shaper and mover of the stage words and pictures.

Looking back at some of his earlier performed works then, the controlling agency of the author is revealed in a clearer light, showing how the theatrical game-plan operating in each play contests any level at which it represents place or character outside the theatre. As Eamonn Jordan comments, McDonagh's Connemara plays 'operate almost totally within the co-ordinates of the dramatic spaces only, almost without reverberation' (2010: 146). McDonagh confuses the signs so that audiences are caught in the headlights with familiar-looking images, while the play arches away from mimesis, back into its own network of devices. More than game-playing postmodernism, a sense of displacement, of baffled disconnection, results.

O'Toole argues that domestic details are pushed into the foreground to make a realistic impact, but they operate more as a satire of merchandising as it appears in lifestyle literature; instead of Gucci or Gaggia, McDonagh's people reach for Complan, Tayto crisps and Kimberley biscuits. The cottage or farmhouse interiors are so semiotically loaded they resemble surrealist still-lives more than a lived-in place. The setting for *The Lonesome West* is a territory divided, crammed with religious figurines, shotgun, crucifix, photo of dog, and orange stove, each object shouting its narrative potential. *A Skull in Connemara* is haunted by theatrical precedents: Beckett's *Waiting for Godot* (the title sourced from Lucky's speech); Shakespeare's Hamlet in Act V, Scene 1, the graveyard; and Synge's *The Playboy of the Western World*, with Christy's resurrected father, whom all thought had been murdered, mirrored by Mairtin's unexpected return in McDonagh's play.

When it comes to destabilising dramatic space, McDonagh uses two particular ways to theatricalise the stage and to unsettle any sure sense of place and any realist frame. First, he interrupts located scenes with the narrative of a letter, read by its author and played in a lit sub-section of the stage. Pato recites his letter to Maureen in Scene 5 of *The Beauty Queen of Leenane* while '[m]ost of the stage is in darkness apart from a spotlight or some such [...] as if in a bedsit in England' (34). Then in complete darkness Pato continues with a letter to his brother, as the audience are jolted out of illusion and are made aware of how, sitting in the gloom, they are in the hands of the playwright and the dramatic cliché on which the structure will turn.

Similarly in both *The Lonesome West* (Scene 5: 'Stage in darkness apart from Welsh' (168)) and *The Cripple of Inishmaan* (Scene 7: 'lights come up on him [Billy] shivering alone on a chair' (74)), the audience sees a lone figure who addresses, as it were, the play itself. In Billy's case there is a twist (so beloved of Katurian in *The Pillowman*) as we learn later that Scene 7 was actually Billy's rehearsal for his film audition, a fiction within a fiction. Elsewhere, scenes set at night emphasise the figures on stage isolated in areas of light while their locations remain undefined.

In his introduction to McDonagh's *Plays: 1*, Fintan O'Toole recognises the playwright's elements of trickery, but frames them in humanist terms as:

bridges over a deep pit of sympathy and sorrow [...] illuminated by a tragic vision of stunted and frustrated lives'.

(1999: xvii)

26

The bridge is an eloquent image of between-ness, of passage, an elsewhere of self and identity. But the sorrow and tragedy are landscapes we gaze at but cannot connect with, destinations at which the plays never quite arrive.

Talking to ourselves alone

Women's voices in Irish theatre have not commonly taken to the monologue form, and for several women playwrights dramatic space is a site of social contest for self-reliance and independence. Stella Feehily's *Duck* (2003) begins and, more significantly, ends with its two young heroines out in public spaces – '*a deserted street*' (3) and '*a roadside*' (109). In between Cat and Sophie pass through the places of family, employment and relationship but in all of these locations they struggle and fail to control what happens. In a spatial *coup de theatre*, three consecutive scenes are set in the bath, where Cat is partnered by her older lover, then by her boyfriend (whose nickname for her is Duck) and lastly is seen chatting with Sophie and then her mother. The interchangeability of the men is signalled in the stage direction introducing the second bath scene: '*Lights snap up. MARK is in the bath where JACK was*' (69). Cat's vulnerability when Mark attacks her brings together the underlying theme of the play, its title, and the role of Sophie, who earlier hints at the semantic context of what happens. Mark 'ducks' Cat, threatening to drown her, re-enacting the medieval or early-modern punishment and social humiliation imposed on women who were considered to be gossiping, disruptive, too much outside the house or otherwise usurping of male authority. In this context, where sub-textual reference is made to women's historicised confinement, spatially and socially, the final image of the play is resistant and theatrically original in an Irish context. Cat and Sophie sit at the roadside, throwing stones in Beckettian mood; they have flown the nest but the play is soberly unresolved on the matter of their path ahead.

Mark O'Rowe's *Howie the Rookie* (1999) centres on two Howies, who both speak their stories from an undefined space. In *Howie* and *Crestfall* (2003) location lies purely in language, which self-consciously maps the marginalised environments of a social underclass. With no connection enacted between characters, all of whom address the audience directly, a profound sense of dislocation and failure of social structures is effected. This is unsettlingly reinforced in the violent, abusive and sometimes funny narratives. Although O'Rowe as a playwright seems very much in love with language (and in *Terminus* (2007) all other stage elements fall well behind it), tragic inevitability in the plays counters the possibilities of speech as utopian: an imaginary route out of social and gender entrapment. *Terminus* (2007) is playful, a violent fantasy shaped into reflexive form so that the audience, who are again addressed directly, are forced to play the part of horrified, fascinated and powerless witness.

O'Rowe's caution with theatricality, although it is held in tension with a highly energised dramatic language, is seen in the dominance of monologue and is visible in a number of Conor McPherson monologue plays. *The Weir* (1997), *Dublin Carol* (2000), *Shining City* (2004) and *The Seafarer* (2006) are set in specific locations represented on stage, but much of McPherson's early work refuses anything more than location through language. With *Come on Over* (2001) the setting comprises two chairs, and the performance context of *Port Authority*, in the same year, is entirely explicit in the opening stage direction: '*The play is set in the theatre*' (McPherson 2004: 132).

McPherson is poetically engaged with the specific geography of the north side of Dublin city, but through solely linguistic reference the locality becomes imaginary and open to participation by the audience. In the featureless matrix of stage emptiness, talk of local pubs, roads and youthful haunts offers a geography of connection while also suggesting the fracturing of the actual places and their residual existence in human memory and identity.

The power of place to express human history and its emotional cargo is theatricalised in recent work by Frank McGuinness, Marina Carr and Enda Walsh. The latter's work shows the audience confined obsessive spaces like psychic crucibles, containing explosive disordered energies. In *The New Electric Ballroom* (premiered Munich 2004) the room in which three women wait is ritually invaded until its transformation into the remembered ballroom opens a possible chink into the future. This quickly slams shut. Behind the room, or within it, the fishing village where the women grew up hovers like a hallucination. The stage space reflects the shape of memory and endless repetition.

This claustrophobic feeling is intensified to an even greater degree in *The Walworth Farce* (2006). Dinny and his sons have left Cork for a dingy flat in London, but their days are devoted to re-playing the family trauma that drove them away in the first place but that they can never escape. This space is psychotic, a projection of deranged obsession. It is a cage made by the past, a bunker dedicated to repetition, against change or the future. Both of Walsh's plays are uncompromisingly theatrical, centred on performativity, deeply playful. The stage austerity of his earlier work such as *Disco Pigs* (1996) and *Bedbound* (2000) has taken a celebratory arc into a dark carnivalesque.

The nouveau riche of the Celtic Tiger era have not made many appearances on Irish stages, but in Marina Carr's *Marble* (2009) their anxieties and dreams disturb the definition of success and aspiration as material. Two couples appear to enjoy the casual privileges of ample disposable income: retrogressive gender roles (women at home; men at the office); and the kind of arrogant self-assurance that had become very recognisable outside the theatre. The scenes take place in vague and banal settings (a restaurant patio, rooms in both houses) but Carr cites Giorgio de Chirico's painting *Melancholy and Mystery of a Street* as encapsulating the mood and landscape 'the near absence of people, the dream shadows, yet full of colour and intrigue' (8). Art confesses to Ben that he has dreamt of Catherine, Ben's wife. Then both Art and Catherine share the same dream of erotic transcendence with one another in a room of marble. The dream devours Catherine and she leaves her family, although she recognises that it is not Art himself, but what he represents that she desires:

> maybe he's just a signal or a beacon, not important in himself but a sign that has brought me to a different place.
>
> (58)

The play proposes overwhelming absorption in an image of the absolute, favoured above all else and to the detriment of all else. The scenes' recognisable social elements (sofas, wine glasses, mobile phones) make no sense against the unseen oneiric realm of irrational passion and impossible cold perfection.

Carr's earlier work, such as *The Mai* (1994), *Portia Coughlan* (1996), *By the Bog of Cats* (1998), *On Raftery's Hill* (2000) and *Ariel* (2002), feature rural settings, and characters who may be monied but who gain little happiness through material prosperity. Hester in *By the Bog of Cats* belongs to the eponymous place as a child belongs to a parent. Her longing for her errant mother's return is so closely identified with the Bog of Cats that she chooses to die rather than leave. Hester's tortured love of place resonates with Synge's lyrical expression of landscape, and both playwrights shadow the beauty and the moody poetry with threat and pain. In *The Mai* and *Portia Coughlan*, the stories (almost monologues) about landscape tell of loss, pain and damage, and The Mai's and Portia's distress mediates the audience's sense of place. Space and place vacillate unstably between the recognisable real and the imaginary symbolic, refusing to allow either to settle and buffeting the characters roughly between desire and unfulfilment.

In both *The Mai* and *Woman and Scarecrow* (2008) Carr uses the idea of the west of Ireland as a utopian space of liberty, fulfilment and also of reckoning. As Yvonne Scott writes in her introduction to the exhibition titled 'The West as Metaphor':

[t]he purity of the national identity was authenticated by the landscape in which it was rooted in turn implying that the native character [...] was both formed by, and analogous to, the environment which supported it.

(Scott 2005: 7)

To be in the west then is a test of authenticity, a measure of identity. In *There Came a Gypsy Riding* (2007) Frank McGuinness clarifies the purpose of the play's west of Ireland setting from the beginning stage direction:

Morning. The magnificent early light of the west of Ireland [...] more threatening, more revealing than electric light could ever be.

(3)

The McKenna family revisits the holiday cottage ('*The time is now.*' [v]) where two years before, their 19 year-old son (?) had killed himself by drowning. An eccentric elderly distant cousin, Bridget, presents them with his suicide note, which she has kept since his death. The space of the play is within the house and outside on the causeway. At several points in the action '*the sea swells*', and there is '*a fierce cry of seabirds*' (22 and 78), and conversations fall frequently into silences. At the end of Act III, '*a blast of wave showers*', the bereaved father (63) who responds as if speaking to the dead boy. McGuinness uses the presence of the sea to counter the rationalisations of the family. They are strangely unsympathetic figures although complexly drawn. The boy's reasons for taking his life are never made clear. The economic success of the father, even in grief, is highlighted, as is the resilience and industry of the mother. The holiday cottage is a sign of their newfound prosperity, but the family moves through the place and quickly abandons it again. It is left to Bridget, who, wheeling a child's buggy, addresses her last lines to the sea or the dead boy:

Don't weep [...] Listen to the rain and the wind. They do the crying. They are your epitaph.

(78)

The play seems to test the family against the place, which is partly embodied by Bridget and haunted by the suicide, and finds the family wanting. Their investment in lives elsewhere and the pragmatic brevity of their stay makes this inevitable. Somehow the questions posed by the boy taking his own life, by the place he chose and by the oddly symbolic presence of Bridget, reflect finally on their lives rather than on his death.

If the dramatic space is fractured, destabilised and refracted, its impact may not always signal negatively. It may also open possibility and outstrip narrative limits, to pose new formations of identity. Anne Hartigan's short play *In Other Worlds* (2003) exploits the mobile phone, and images of medical technology and the body, to explore relationship and space in a way that makes altogether virtual the issue of place. Presence becomes a function of sound, language and light on stage, as the audience visualise the imagined location of the central character, whose body is visibly being kept alive by a respirator.

Perhaps one of the most complex explorations of identity and place in Irish theatre is achieved by Anne Devlin in *After Easter* (1994). The scene opens with Greta, '*a spotlight on her face as she speaks*' (1) and the sound of a bus screeching to a halt. Greta's location is revealed only later, when the shadowy figure that has been in the background comes forward and turns out to be a psychiatrist. This uncertainty of borders within the performance space of the play as a whole is a consistent element throughout. Greta's quest for identity sees her negotiate the borders of Irishness and Englishness, Catholic spirituality, family bereavement and reconciliation. The ending of the play opens it out in a very remarkable way, bringing together an image of motherhood with a narrative that points towards self and identity as centred in finding a voice that is uninhibited by inherited myths and structures, whether national or otherwise, and points towards an unfamiliar spaciousness:

And he took me to a place where the rivers come from, where you come from [...] and this is my own story.

(75)

The dramatic spaces in Irish plays seem to reflect and to question the pressures on place as a context for identity, the human reliance on it and its changing configurations in the globalised and technologised world we occupy. If there is a sense of loss and disorder in many Irish plays, is it a loss of nation or a setting of terms for an encounter with uncertainty?

Does globalisation mean the destruction of place as meaningful? Can place maintain its value, freed from nation? Can the theatre of a small nation maintain its value if the small nation effectively no longer exists?

Works cited

Benson, C. (2001), *The Cultural Psychology of Self*, London: Routledge.

Carr, M. (2009), *Marble*, Oldcastle: Gallery Books.

——— (1999), *Plays: 1: Low in the Dark, The Mai, Portia Coughlan, By the Bog of Cats*, London: Faber.

Casey, E. S. (1993), *Getting Back Into Place*, Bloomington: Indiana University Press.

Devlin, A. (1994), *After Easter*, London: Faber.

Feehily, S. (2003), *Duck*, London: Nick Hern Books.

Friel, B. (1984), *Selected Plays of Brian Friel*, London: Faber.

Hartigan, A. (2003), *In Other Worlds*, Unpublished Manuscript.

Hughes, D. (2000), 'Who the Hell Do We Think We Still Are? Reflections on Irish Theatre and Identity', in Eamonn Jordan (ed.), *Theatre Stuff*, Dublin: Carysfort Press.

Hynes, G. (2001), 'Interview with Cathy Leeney', in Lilian Chambers [et al.] (ed.), *Theatre Talk*, Dublin: Carysfort Press.

Jordan, E. (2010), *Dissident Dramaturgies*, Dublin: Irish Academic Press.

Kiberd, D. (1996), *Inventing Ireland*, London: Vintage.

Lonergan, P. (2009), *Theatre and Globalization: Irish Drama in the Celtic Tiger Era*, Basingstoke: Palgrave Macmillan.

McAuley, G. (1999), *Space in Performance: Making Meaning in Theatre*, Ann Arbor: University of Michigan Press.

McDonagh, M. (1998), *The Cripple of Inishmaan*, New York: Vintage International.

——— (2003), *The Pillowman*, London: Faber.

——— (1999), *Plays: 1: The Beauty Queen of Leenane, A Skull in Connemara, The Lonesome West*, introduction by Fintan O'Toole, London: Methuen.

McGuinness, F. (2007), *There Came a Gypsy Riding*, London: Faber.

McPherson, C. (2004), *Plays: Two*, London: Nick Hern Books.

O'Toole, F. (2003), *After the Ball*, Dublin: New Island.

O'Rowe, M. (1999), *Howie the Rookie*, London: Nick Hern Books.

Scott, Y. (2005), 'Introduction', *The West as Metaphor*, Dublin: Royal Hibernian Academy.

Walsh, E. (2008), *The New Electric Ballroom*, London: Nick Hern Books.

——— (2007), *The Walworth Farce*, London: Nick Hern Books.

Note

1 All stage directions are presented in italics.

Chapter 2

Processes and Interactive Events: Theatre and Scottish Devolution

Ian Brown

Any study of the impact of events runs the danger of reifying individual dates as watersheds. More often events and their dates are best understood as marking the flow of currents through time, rather than being seen as absolute moments of singular significance. Certainly, a battle on a given day may be decisive, but in itself it results from long processes and creates new ones. If that is true of an event like a battle, how much more is it of a development like Scottish devolution? It may have been Ron Davis as Welsh Secretary who in January 1998 launched in Parliament the famous dictum: 'Devolution is a process, not an event'. In Scotland the late Donald Dewar is regularly credited with it. Though others have disputed he said this, he certainly said things like this in the late 1990s (Macwhirter 2007). This chapter argues that, just as devolution is a process, and a long-term one at that, so are the complex interactions of theatre and devolution. It argues that devolution and the 1999 re-establishment of the Scottish Parliament changed 'Scotland' and theatre reflected that. It also argues that theatre, in common with other artforms, had an interactive impact on devolution. Sam Galbraith, then Minister for the Arts in the new Scottish government, addressing the 1999 Edinburgh Festival seminar of arts organisations, asserted that, in his view, the artists had made devolution possible. To understand what Galbraith implies, we need to understand the interaction of the devolutionary process and theatre (and the arts in general) as continuous, traceable even to before the 1979 referendum (when a positive vote for Scottish devolution fell below a voting threshold), let alone that of 1997. Perhaps, indeed the impact of the arts as identified by Galbraith is particularly intense in a relatively small nation like Scotland with its own broadcasting and news institutions, history and cultural formations. This may be especially so when the community of the nation, of 'the realm of Scotland' – to use an ancient Scottish constitutional term – is debating its future within a larger multi-national state whose apparent unity has from its negotiated beginning in 1707 included guarantees for separate Scottish law, established religion, education and other civic functions. The impact of these institutions, in addition to that of Scotland's languages – Scots and Gaelic as well as English – all interact with cultural manifestations to both interrogate and celebrate difference within the apparently United Kingdom.

The impetus that led to the 1979 referendum followed the surge of political support for the Scottish National Party after the 1967 Hamilton by-election when its first peacetime Member of Parliament, Winifred Ewing, was elected. The subsequent discovery of oil in the North Sea off Scotland provided an economic background to the rise of support for the idea of separate governance for Scotland. All of this accompanied the beginnings of what is now widely seen as a Scottish theatrical renaissance, starting some time between the opening of the Traverse Theatre in 1963 and the foundation of the Scottish Society of Playwrights in 1973. This in some ways drew on the experiments and creative achievements of the mid-twentieth century Scottish Literary Renaissance led by such figures as Hugh MacDiarmid. A key element in 1970s theatre was rediscovery and theatrical exploitation of Scots language's resources. In the 1920s the miner-playwright Joe Corrie had used Scots for political plays, including *In Time o Strife* set during the 1926 General Strike, before making his living in the 1930s from writing comedies. From that decade, Robert MacLellan and Alexander Reid used Scots in historical dramas. Their motivation, Katja Lenz has observed, 'may lie in its usability as a vehicle for asserting the national culture, for marking it off from the English or the joint British one, by demonstrating the existence of a separate history' (Lenz 1996: 309). Meanwhile Scots was widely used in comedies, largely the couthy, that is to say 'cosy' or 'folksy', one-act comedies popularised by members of the Scottish Community Drama Association (founded in 1926). In the 1940s, 1950s and 1960s, Robert Kemp's and, then, Victor Carin's highly successful Scots translations of classic comedies by Molière, Goldoni and von Kleist appeared. Meanwhile, for a period after the War, Glasgow Unity Theatre produced a series of dramas in Scots concerned with social conditions, predating the work of the 1950s English kitchen-sink playwrights. By 1970 there was a large body of work, almost all comedy, available in Scots. The sea change in the 1970s was that playwrights began, following the intermittent exemplars of Corrie and the Unity playwrights, to use the language for a wider range of more serious topics.

The way creative writers use Scots is seen in Scottish literary-linguistic criticism as having very particular social and political implications. In 1988, for example, Derrick McClure observed:

[In the eighteenth century] English was considered a more polite language than Scots. To write in Scots, therefore, was an act with overt and inescapable cultural, even political, implications: a deliberate gesture of support for a denigrated tongue.

(McClure 1988: 37)

In 1991 he further commented:

any piece of writing in Scots is an ideological statement, a proclamation that the writer is refusing to be identified with the politically and culturally dominant English-speaking community.

(McClure 1991: 195)

In 1999 Katja Lenz added:

The decision to write a play in Scots is still a political step. With some authors, the choice of Scots is clearly a statement of national and cultural politics. In less radical cases, Scots serves to transmit a feeling of specifically Scottish identity.

(Lenz 1999: 352)

At the very least, as John Corbett put it in the same year, '[t]he value-systems according to language varieties are culturally relative' (Corbett 1999: 9). In other words, there is a clear critical consensus about the politico-cultural implications of using Scots in literature or theatre. Liz Lochhead's 1984 comment shows a writer agreeing:

> I do like to use Glasgow and West of Scotland register, but that's only because it's part of my own childhood and private register that I know intimately. I'm certainly interested in Scottishness, but I feel that the territory that gets delineated is a macho William McIlvanney and Tom Leonard world and that's what Glasgowness feeds into.
>
> (quoted in Brown 1984: 18–19)

Two things emerge from Lochhead's comment. Firstly, as with McClure, Lenz and Corbett, she recognises that the use of Scots on stage is profoundly linked with the assertion of Scottishness, of cultural and political identity. Secondly, speaking in 1984, she sees that language as somehow linked with West Coast machismo. In this, she reflects the phenomenon that Carla Sassi in 2009 summarised as 'the powerful literary strain that rigidly connotes Scottish nationhood as male, working-class and, ideologically, as socialist or republican' (Sassi 2009: 152–153).

These perceptions are surely derived particularly from 1970s literature, and especially drama, leading up to the 1979 referendum. Major masculinised, West Coast, urban, often workplace, plays include Bill Bryden's *Willie Rough* (1972), Tom Buchan's *The Great Northern Welly Boot Show* (1972), Roddy McMillan's *The Bevellers* (1973), Hector Macmillan's *The Rising* (1973), Tom McGrath's *The Hard Man* (1977) and John Byrne's *The Slab Boys* trilogy (1978, 1979, 1982). Not all that decade's drama fitted this mould. While some of John McGrath's work for 7:84 (Scotland) might do so, *The Cheviot, The Stag and the Black Black Oil* (1973) clearly has other foci. Donald Campbell's and Stewart Conn's plays deal with different aspects of Scotland, though even their work is often concerned with male-focused issues, like the Leith-born mercenary imprisoned in Africa in Conn's *Play Donkey* (1977). Perhaps only McGrath's *Little Red Hen* (1975), Robert David MacDonald's *Summit Conference* (1978) and Campbell's *The Widows of Clyth* (1979) show male playwrights allowing women central roles. The present author's *Mary* (1977) is arguably different, being driven by a central historical figure. What all the plays – except perhaps MacDonald's – show, however, is a concern with what it is to be Scottish, the particularities of the Scottish experience and assertion of the value and richness of Scottish identities. In the 1970s, though, by and large these identities are expressed in masculinised forms.

Meantime, what had been a rather limited dramatic tradition in the Gaelic-language community, only established outside folk drama expressions in the twentieth century, developed through the 1960s and 1970s, through playwrights like Tormod Calum Dòmhnallach, Fionnlagh MacLeòid (Finlay Macleod), Donaidh MacIlleathain (Donnie Maclean) and Iain Moireach. Michelle MacLeod and Moray Watson have identified Iain Crichton Smith as a key figure:

Like many of this era's plays, his eschew traditional boundaries and explore wide-ranging topics; sometimes they are humorous; sometimes they concern serious issues, like the betrayal of Christ in *An Coileach* (*The Cockerel*, 1966) or the Clearances and human conscience in *A' Chùirt* (*The Court*, 1966).

(MacLeod and Watson 2007: 281–282)

They also identify European, Absurdist influences on the period's Gaelic drama. While much of this drama was inaccessible to non-Gaelic speakers, it contributed to a wider perception of the potential multivalency of what 'Scottish' could be in a modern age. It also emphasised the diversity of what constituted the 'small' nation of Scotland. It drew, as did some Scots-language theatre, on Irish examples. The examples lay not so much in the language choices a Scot might make, for Irish drama followed O'Connell's nineteenth century lead in appropriating the language of colonial power, English. Rather, they lay in their assertion, in the plays of Yeats or Synge, for example, of the otherness of the small nations in the British archipelago and their historical and cultural concerns. For Scots these were often expressed precisely through what was seen as empowering language choices and non-unionist or non-Anglicised perspectives. Smith himself, quoted by MacLeod and Watson, identified this sense of a wider outlook:

Some years ago I wrote a play in Gaelic about the Trojan War and it was felt by some that this was not a suitable topic for a Gaelic writer. I disagreed and still disagree. There is no reason why the Gaelic writer, if he wishes, should not comment on ideas and events which transcend the Gaelic world.

(cited in Macleod and Watson 2007: 281)

In 1978, a Gaelic theatre company, Fir Chlis ('Merry Dancers' – lit. 'agile men' – or 'Northern Lights'), was established, though it lasted only three years. Nonetheless, the expressive potential of Scottish drama in the years up to the first devolution referendum was being challenged and developed not by Scots- and English-language playwrights alone.

Despite the 1979 referendum's majority for an Assembly, it failed to deliver one: what was widely seen as gerrymandering required a threshold vote beyond a simple majority. The result caused dismay, but did not halt Scottish theatre's dynamic or its interaction with devolutionary thinking. After 1979 new vital currents asserted the Scottish body politic's vibrancy and wide-ranging nature. The already-developing revitalisation of Scottish theatre broadened, accelerated and strengthened. A key element was the emergence of several leading women playwrights. As is clear from the names above, there had been a male-dominated repertoire, with only the Unity playwright Ena Lamont Stewart, Joan Ure from the 1960s on and Marcella Evaristi from the mid-1970s achieving lasting prominence. The revival of Stewart's *Men Should Weep* (1947), partly rewritten, as part of 7:84 (Scotland)'s 1982 *Clydebuilt* season, marked it as a classic text, while others new to playwriting found wider and wider theatrical acceptance. Partly this arose from feminist initiatives of the 1960s and 1970s, but it also arose from the fact that over the centuries Scottish women had contributed importantly to other literary genres. Indeed, in the theatre, Joanna Baillie had been at the end of the eighteenth century arguably the most important Scottish playwright. Whatever masculinisation had taken over in the early twentieth century in drama, women writers were still important in other forms. It may be no surprise that one of the first of the new women playwrights, Liz Lochhead, was already, before writing drama, a widely admired poet. Alongside her, Sue Glover, Anne-Marie di Mambro, Sharman Macdonald and Anne Downie emerged as important playwrights in the 1980s followed later by others like Rona Munro, Isobel Wright and Zinnie Harris. The male-centredness Sassi observed was passé as they rejected 1970s masculinisation, claiming the stage for their dramaturgy, themes and language. Their arrival heralded a new generation of 1980s and 1990s male playwrights, including Peter Arnott, John (now Jo) Clifford, David Greig, David Harrower and Stephen Greenhorn. New writers – like Chris Hannan in his particularly women-focussed plays *Elizabeth Gordon Quinn* (1985), set during the First World War, and *Shining Souls* (1996) – explored the delusions and aspirations of working-class Glaswegians in different less male-centred ways from the 1970s generation. Yet that generation, in the work of Tom McGrath or John Byrne, for example, continued to develop. The work of Byrne – both in the theatre, where the segments of *The Slab Boys* trilogy have regularly been revived, and in his television dramas, *Tutti Frutti* (1988) and *Your Cheatin' Heart* (1990) – paved the way for some of the most exciting contemporary Scottish drama. His work juxtaposes the world of international popular culture with that of the local, setting both in a lively creative loop of inter-reference and intertextuality. All these playwrights explored fresh issues and the possibilities of a new Scottish drama, and so those of a new Scottish politics. It is as if the shock of the outcome of the 1979 referendum triggered a radical revision of thinking about what Scotland, its societies, communities and identities were and could be. Throughout the 1980s radical alternatives – and less macho versions of maleness – were explored. Arguably the Scottish parliament represents an effort to achieve a revisited national politics, while affecting and shaping anew Scotland's place in the world, a small nation finding sister communities in, say, Quebec, Malawi, Catalunya or Croatia. Similarly Scottish dramatists have powerfully explored the interaction and, sometimes, conflict between international and national culture.

This international outlook was reinforced by the fact that the refreshed Scottish theatre was more diverse than that of the 1970s, not only in foregrounding women and younger playwrights, but also in featuring a surge of important contemporary translations. John Corbett has observed:

> It is significant that the two great periods of translation into Scots – the sixteenth and twentieth centuries – have been times when the process of national refashioning was at its most urgent.

(Corbett 1999: 7)

Liz Lochhead's *Tartuffe* (1985) and Edwin Morgan's *Cyrano de Bergerac* (1992) were landmarks, bringing French classics into vibrant Glaswegian-inflected Scots, full of fresh linguistic vim and sharp, satirical register shifts, using Scots to deflate pomposity and assert a demotic dynamic and dynamic demotic. As a maid sees off her importuner, Lochhead rhymes 'randy' and 'houghmagandie' (Scots for sexual activity). Morgan offers us a Muse with unpretentious language:

You and the Muse are total strangers, but
If you did happen tae meet, she'd stoap yer strut.
She'd scunner, fatso, at yer wobblin fruit,
And kick yer backside wi her classic boot

Important as these translations were, the leading ones were those by Bill Findlay and Martin Bowman from Quebecois, mainly of Michel Tremblay's plays, in a stunning series of nine premières, from *The Guid Sisters* (1989) to *If Only …* (2002). Mark Fisher in *The Guardian* (29 October 1992) described Tremblay as the 'best playwright Scotland never had'. Translations from Quebecois had a particular politico-cultural impact: Tremblay was writing out of another national community within a larger political entity, with its own language and identity issues. The experience of Scotland was clearly not unique. Findlay and Bowman helped internationalise Scottish perceptions of its political identity. And Tremblay's themes derived from conceptions of community and sexuality that escaped a dominant male, workplace version of society, reinforced the lively work of the women playwrights and gay playwrights like John Binnie and Christopher Deans. Binnie in such plays as *Accustomed to Her Face* (1993) explored the excitements, rewards, sorrows and dignity of same sex love and growth to emotional and sexual maturity. Deans in plays like *Molly's Collar and Tie* (1996) and *Smells and Bells* (1998) brought his own sharp insight and ribald humour to his themes. The latter attracted particular censure from some quarters for its cheerful depiction of male fellatio in the confessional. Jackie Kay's *Chiaroscuro* (1986) dealt with four characters whose friendship is challenged and strengthened by experience of racism, sexism and homophobia. Grace Barnes approached Shetland experience writing in Shetlandic in *Wir Midder da Sea* (1999).

Playwrights were redefining the nation. Scottish theatre's vitality in the devolutionary decades was a key expression, and determinant, of national cultural and political identity, or to be more precise, identities. Those were inclusive, male and female, beyond and within the Central Belt, island and mainland, heterosexual, homosexual, bisexual, and transsexual, Scots, English and Gaelic – Tosg ('Ambassador') Theatre Company was established in 1996 (though it closed in 2007, when its founder, Simon MacKenzie, fell seriously ill, dying prematurely in 2008).

For dramatists, as for all twentieth-century Scottish writers, the uses of language and theatrical diversity were important elements in addressing the history and ideology of the Scottish experience and the nature of Scotland, Scottish history and Scottishness itself. John McGrath was key here, his *Joe's Drum* (1979) an early reaction to the disappointment of the 1979 result. Complementing his developed theatrical style, he created expansive productions, exploring larger constitutional issues and Scotland's historic relations, in big spaces like Glasgow's Tramway Theatre (*Border Warfare*, 1989) and Edinburgh's International Conference Centre (*Ane Satire of the Four Estates*, 1996). Indeed the latter title marks his long historical perspective, reflecting Sir David Lindsay's epic sixteenth-century *Ane Satyre of the Thrie Estaitis*. Bill Bryden had revived that great comic dissection of bad and good governance in 1973. He himself wrote – and directed in the Engine Shed of the former Govan shipyard, Harland and Wolff – vast populist shows revisiting formative moments for modern Scotland. *The Ship* (1990) dramatised the building of the QE2; *The Big Picnic* (1994), Scottish soldiers' World War One experiences. Theatre's varied languages were part of its strength, like that of songwriters like The Proclaimers (the twins Craig and Charlie Reid, who write largely in Scots English and sing in their unmodified Leith accents) or Runrig (whose rock music incorporates from time to time bagpipes and Gaelic lyrics). In a culture with broadcasting largely dominated by London and North American voices, Scots not only were heard, but asserted themselves. Their own accents, themes and approach to international issues re-echoed the sense of a separate value system requiring its own democratic expression, redefining it in ways which, in the end, were reflected in the Scottish parliament's differences from Westminster. Holyrood's proportional representation has broken London's Labour and Conservative two-party dominance, in a way that even the Conservative-dominated Lib-Con Westminster 2010 coalition does not. Agendas driven by very different cultural and economic drivers than 1970s theatre's male working classes – environmentalism, gender, sexuality, region and, indeed, the nation itself – have found expression in varieties impossible in traditional Westminster politics, even in the days of the Cameron-Clegg coalition. This still appears to think and work in terms of a Parliament of opposition rather than the diversity and gradations of view inherent in the fan-shaped Scottish parliamentary chamber designed by a Catalonian, Enric Miralles. The range of party membership of the Scottish Parliament as first elected in 1999 – six parties plus two independents – reflected one form of the various Scottish self-confident identities there could be. That range, which makes Scottish parliamentary politics so difficult for the dominant UK parties to manage, was already seen in and nurtured by playwrights' Scottish (and international) dramatic explorations from the 1970s on. After 1979, the concept of Scotland expressed in drama had become more complex, wide-ranging, multivalent and full of difference. It reflected, supported and reinforced the developing sense of identity and self-confidence that allowed the parliament's election and its party-political complexity, something partly echoed in the multilingual, coalition-based experience of the Welsh Assembly. It helped develop and shape a sense of national community/communities and interacted with the politico-cultural impetus that, within two decades, brought two referenda and the Scottish parliament's reopening. If such a claim seems inflated, one need only remember the witness of Sam Galbraith, a senior and, by reputation, very hard-nosed politician.

Yet, though a fundamental thesis of this chapter is that the devolutionary settlement is part of a process, not the product of an event, the Scottish Parliament's re-establishment is an event that has impinged on twenty-first century Scottish theatre. Part of that impact, as well as the forces leading to it, may be seen in the poem by Iain Crichton Smith, poet-playwright in Gaelic, Scots and English, read as part of the Parliament's opening ceremony:

Let our three-voiced country
Sing in a new world
Joining the other rivers without dogma,
But with friendliness to all around her.

Let her new river shine on a day
That is fresh and glittering and contemporary;

Let it be true to itself and to its origins
Inventive, original, philosophical,
Its institutions mirror its beauty;
Then without shame we can esteem ourselves.

The poem's title, 'The Beginning of a New Song (for the opening of the Scottish Parliament, 1999)', confirms the sense that the continuities under discussion, running into and from the Parliament's reopening, overlie much deeper continuities. It is a clear intertextual reference to a famous remark of the unionist Earl of Seafield, Chancellor of Scotland. In 1707, he signed the Treaty of Union and so ended – as he thought for ever – Scotland's ancient Parliament and sovereign independence, saying, 'There's ane end of ane auld sang'. Seafield's Scots is echoed and revisited by the Gaelic poet-playwright Smith's English, emphasising values which Smith sees as key to the identity of the Scotland(s) he – no doubt idealistically – imagines: multivoiced (and so multivalent), singing and new, undogmatic and international, fresh and contemporary with regard to inventiveness, originality and philosophy. Above all, Smith imagines 'our' – note the inclusive communal word – 'three-voiced country' esteeming itself. Such self-esteem was a reassertion of the value and resistant identities of Scottish communities and ideas within the Union settlement, whose post-war forms and structures leading thinkers in the 1980s and 1990s argued had led people in Scotland into inferiorist self-limiting perceptions of their nation and selves, a 'cringe'. Key texts in this dialogue arguing for a more balanced, moderate sense of national identities within international perspectives were produced by, for example, Craig Beveridge and Ronald Turnbull (1989) and Cairns Craig (1996). Those identities were developed by earlier playwriting and reinforced by that which came after 1999.

In this, David Greig is a key figure who is now translated into and produced in over 30 languages. His *One Way Street* (1995) explored mainland European experience, while *The Architect* (1996) examined the growing pressures on a young Edinburgh man, faced by the compromises of received social values. In both, Greig dramatised the tensions of a middle class whose European perspectives and material success cannot redress emotional sterility. Greig enjoys experiment, reflecting the variety of Scotland's new political settlements, still open-ended and in process. *Caledonia Dreaming* (1997) was being written as the event it concerned, the 1997 UK General Election, was under way. Its diverse plot-lines, all including a running gag concerning the rumoured presence of Sean Connery in Edinburgh as the new UK settlement was being decided, embodied disparate possibilities for Scotland in a post-election UK. The children's play *Danny 306 + Me (4 Ever)* (1999) requires human and puppet performers. *The Speculator* (1999) returns to history, exploring the proto-Thatcherite career of the Scots banker, visionary and fraud, John Law, trying to introduce paper money in eighteenth-century France, with disastrous consequences, including economic collapse. *Outlying Islands* (2002), driven by sexuality and jealousy, and *8000 Metres* (2004), which involved actors performing in climbing ropes, investigate more intimate themes of human relationship and personal identity. Such theatrical experiment continues: Greig's *The Strange Undoing of Prudencia Hart* (2011) draws on the traditions of Scottish Border ballads in a rhymed text performed in a pub, supposedly after hours. Meanwhile his work as a co-founder of the experimental and cross-artform company Suspect Culture (1993–2009) includes *One-Two* (2003). This investigates the rhythms at the core of human existence and beyond words, the sounds of music and of heartbeat, through a complex interaction of instruments and characters. Greig has sustained a formal experimental strand in his work and he even appears as a named character in his own *San Diego* (2003) where innovative form sustains fabulous invention of the disenfranchised and emotionally lost in the transitory worlds of California. Greig's dramaturgical approach is collaborative, including his 'play with songs', written with Gordon McIntyre, *Midsummer* (2009), where again boundaries are for crossing. One of the key dimensions for theatre, and literature in general, arising in the last decade is the ways in which Scotland conceives of itself as 'Scotlands', multilingual, varied and intercultural both historically and contemporaneously. Several critical commentators address this issue, including Douglas Gifford (2007), the present author with Colin Nicolson (Brown and Nicholson 2007) and Carla Sassi (2009). Greig, like many of his generation and as such commentators observe, seeks what devolution continues to allow, what the present author has called 'Reconfiguration of the Possible'.

Greig is part of a new wave of Scottish theatre writing – experimental in style and focused on 'marginal' groups within Scottish society – which has gathered momentum since the 1997 referendum. Two key texts of that year mark that period's beginning. David Harrower's *Knives in Hens* (1997) presents the complex politics of illicit male-female love in a primal rural context. While he does not write here in Scots, the rhythms of his speech are attenuated and Scots-accented. Harrower's play, now produced across the world, explores within individual psychopathologies the emotional drives that cause the woman to find love away from her husband and with the sensual miller. Their actions' transgression is powerfully conveyed in tense dialogue, where boundaries are refused and new emotional resolutions sought. Stephen Greenhorn's *Passing Places* (1997) mimics the road movie form. His protagonists make a pilgrimage from the post-industrial world of Central Scotland – the typical 1970s play location, now shorn of workplaces in which drama might be set – through the Highlands with a surfboard taken in lieu of a debt, which, unknown to them, contains a drug stash. Pursued by the drugs' owner, bent on vengeance, they encounter along the way the myths by which both Lowland and Highland Scotland have been represented. Greenhorn's Highlands are not full of couthy crofters, but of rather unexpected cultural entrepreneurs and settlers. The accents of contemporary Scotland are varied, and include committed inhabitants of Scotland whose birth and voices are English. Greenhorn's humour and vitality is typical of a generation of playwrights for whom Scotland is neither a lost cause to elegise nor potential utopia. Rather like the surfboard the *Passing Places* protagonists carry, it is a nexus in which international cultural symbols are constantly juxtaposed with the realities of life in a relatively small, and often liminal, community. The play ends in Thurso, an unexpected, but genuine, surfing Mecca, where the board, potentially an emblem of freedom and easy escapism, is revealed as corrupted by its contents. One of the heroes is ready to travel further, expanding his identity outwards; the other returns home, enlarged by his experience and ready to participate in a renewed and redefined Scotland.

Both Greenhorn and Harrower have gone to further exploratory work. Greenhorn's next play, *Dissent* (1998) was concerned with the career and compromises of an aspirant Member of the Scottish Parliament in the new post-devolution settlement. Even before the parliament was established, it was subject to cross-examination and the motives of its potential participants questioned. Greenhorn also developed the conception of, and in 2002 launched, *River City*, BBC Scotland's long-running soap. This, after a somewhat rocky start, has established itself as a regular feature of Scottish popular television drama. Greenhorn's exploration of genre crossover continued with his musical *Sunshine on Leith* (2007), taking the music from The Proclaimers eponymous second album (1988) to show love, loss, exile and return from exile among modern Scots. Harrower continues voyaging through human emotions' bleaker side. *Dark Earth* (2003) examined modern tensions between urban and rural, modern and atavistic in the shadow of the Antonine Wall. Set in the shadow of the Roman attempt to contain an older generation of people living in what is now Scotland, the play could not more clearly visualise a dramaturgical structure questioning the nature of current Scottish identities. *Blackbird* (2005) continues his examination of emotional conflict and boundary transgression. Its middle-aged hero, Ray, is visited by Una, now 27, with whom fifteen years earlier he had an affair. He has re-established himself on prison release under a new name, but she has tracked him down. She struggles to understand her emotional turmoil and ambiguous feelings. Ray does not know how to react, fending her off. Both give an impression of remaining mutually attracted. In a chilling intervention, a young girl enters for a moment and behaves towards Ray in a manner suggesting a repetition of his involvement with underage girls. Like *Knives in Hens*, this play has been translated and performed across the world. In searching the murky regions of the psyche, Harrower both revisits the determinism and dualism of a *Justified Sinner* (James Hogg, 1824) or *Jekyll and Hyde* (Robert Louis Stevenson, 1886) and creates a universalised metaphor, like these, for humanity's sometimes unspeakable desires and demands.

Scottish playwrights since the turn of the century have, like Greig and Greenhorn in their different ways, been fascinated by the potential of theatrical genre-transgression. Some have developed in perhaps unexpected ways. Anthony Neilson, for example, first came to notice in the 1990s, being defined, perhaps reductively, as one of the, in Aleks Sierz's terms, 'in-yer-face' school. Alongside other younger playwrights like Sarah Kane and Mark Ravenhill, his plays were seen as often violent and shocking, exploring dark aspects of society and human nature. Certainly, his earlier plays are dark and sometimes horrific. *Normal: the Dusseldorf Ripper* (1991) starkly portrays a murderer's mind. *Penetrator* (1993) examines the male psyche's beastlier aspects. *The Censor* (1997), its main characters an actress in porn films and a film censor, attacks hypocritical values through direct language and action, including onstage defecation. *Stitching* (2002) shows physical and emotional abuse's impact in a collapsing marriage. Here, the audience faces several stomach-churning moments detailing the self-abuse that such relationships may produce, one of the stitchings the title concerns being the heroine's attempts to sew up her own vaginal entrance. Yet, in the same year, his *Edward Gant's Amazing Feats of Loneliness* was produced. Here Neilson achieves a theatrical magic realism, in which Edward Gant presents the audience with performance and metaperformance. Based on the Victorian fascination with freak shows, and full of bad-taste jokes of remarkable hilarity, Neilson explores the freakishness of the human heart and mind through vivid theatrical imagery. He uses puppets and surreal characters – like a young woman whose face is ravaged by pimples from which seep miraculous pearls (and whose husband leaves her for an oyster) – to shape a vivid theatrical language and create an outré world of fantastic imagination. *The Wonderful World of Dissocia* (2004) again reimagines the world and reconfigures the possible with zany humour and deep compassion. Through his heroine, Lisa, and her personal world, Dissocia, he explores the ambivalent nature of mental illness. The first act takes place in the wildly surreal colourful world of the subject's mind. At times scary, it is mostly full of colour and fun, exciting and vital, peopled from her imagination by eccentric Alice-in-Wonderland characters. The second act sees the patient silent and drugged in a hospital's sterile black-and-white surroundings, where carers and family struggle to understand her as she finds the prospect of becoming well on their terms rather unattractive. They want her to leave Dissocia, whereas she wants to be at home and embraced. Neilson presents a compelling and often very funny alternative world of ambivalent values and unreliable perceptions. He is clear about his playwriting's wellspring and place in a changing Scottish repertoire. At the 2005 Gateway Theatre gathering of playwrights, he linked his writing to earlier Scottish drama. He referred to his parents' acting in Donald Campbell's historical play, *The Jesuit* (1976), claiming that experience of rehearsals taught him early about intertwining the personal, emotional and theatrical. Neilson takes tired reality and exposes its hidden depths. In *Realism* (2006), his hero, Stuart McQuarrie, played at the première by the actor Stuart McQuarrie, is seen in an everyday, mundane, domestic setting while around him and drawing him in are the vibrant and fantastic surreal images, dreams and desires underlying and infusing apparently boring reality. We see Stuart and, at the same time, what is happening inside his head. He can, for example, answer *Any Questions?* as it is broadcast. He has a cat that treats him with acutely observed, exquisitely funny and surly contempt. In his mind, he can drop his girl friend, be as rude as he likes to cold-callers and conjure up a chorus line to dance through the stage of his room. His inner life extrudes and explodes around him. In the final scene, when we return to a domestic scene in which his unhappy relations with his girlfriend are clear, we are left with the knowledge that the most tedious everyday existence may be counterpart to a spectacular emotional and mental life. Neilson in the 1990s may have written 'in-yer-face', but in the new century he has brought perceptions of a magical, even magical realist, potential to reshape the world and the way we see it.

While Neilson works in English, two other younger male playwrights, Douglas Maxwell and Gregory Burke, have used demotic Scots. Both have produced landmark works with specific directors and companies. Maxwell's *Decky does a Bronco* (2000) was directed by Ben Harrison of Grid Iron Theatre Company, which experiments with productions grown out of a wide variety of specific sites. Maxwell's open-air play takes place in a children's swing park where an older man, David, recalls the events of the summer of 1983 in Girvan, an Ayrshire seaside town. Its title refers to a trick young people perform on swings. Maxwell describes it:

> To bronco a swing you stand on it, work up to the bumps, level with the bar, kick the swing over your head and jump beneath it. It looks ace and makes a hell of a racket.
>
> (Maxwell 2000)

A bronco combines adventure and vandalism (the swing chains end up spun tightly round the bar, unusable till someone manages to untangle them). The play builds round the bantering relationships of eight nine-year-old boys, played by adults, and their adult memories, while Decky, who has never been able to do a bronco, never appears. At the end of a play full of humour, and the physical sight of the actors playing on the swings and doing broncos, we learn Decky, the smallest one, fell victim to a murderous paedophile. The play is full of irony and innocence lost, the production original and the dialogue and language lively. Maxwell constantly continues to seek experimental boundaries to push. *Variety* (2002), about variety's decline and presented in Edinburgh's King's Theatre, once a major variety hall, did not quite succeed, ironically given its venue, in fully theatricalising its topic. *Helmet* (2002), about Playstation games, however, uses their imagery and language within the electronic theatrical world of the play itself. The action of *If Destroyed True* (2005) unfolds in front of a giant computer screen and chat room messages as sinister authorities seek to maintain New Flood's title as the 'Worst Town in Scotland'. There we see family fragmentation, the death of the hero's drug-addicted mother – and later that of his gay lover when their virtual relationship is violated – and his reconciliation with his once-estranged grandmother. Burke, meantime, in at least two of his plays has explored the possibilities of a powerful Scots, based closely on his native Fife dialect. *Gagarin Way* (2001) uses it to explore the unlikely comedic potential of a factory heist gone agley, its muscular dialogue, typical of contemporary Scottish drama. He presents a specific Scottish experience and explores, simultaneously, questions of globalisation and corruption. His greatest success to date is *Black Watch* (2006). This combines the recruiting social context in Fife (home with Tayside of the Black Watch regiment), experiences of the Iraq War through Jocks' eyes and a summary history of the regiment and its processes of developing – and sometimes betraying back home – *esprit de corps*. Under John Tiffany's direction for the National Theatre of Scotland (NTS), it melds words, dance, movement, music, lighting and sound design into a transverse production of startling impact. Theatrical imagination and linguistic vitality (swearing moves beyond obscenity into a profane poetics) achieve a powerful synthesis as Burke uses interviews with former soldiers for a particular version of authenticity. The play has won awards and plaudits worldwide. It has also, and rightly, been criticised for unquestioning acceptance of the ethos of militaristic regimentalism, and for chauvinism in one *coup de théâtre*, the blowing up of a group of soldiers, in failing to include an Iraqi interpreter's death in the original episode (Archibald 2008: 8–13).

Meantime, two women playwrights, Liz Lochhead and her younger colleague Zinnie Harris have this century moved in contrasting new ways. Lochhead has followed her first translation, *Tartuffe* (1985), with a flurry of five new translations since 2000, engaging with international playwriting in exciting and catholic ways, recasting possibilities for post-1999 Scottish theatre and its exploitation of translation. Her *Medea* (2000) (presented within a trilogy, *The Greeks*, with Greig's *Oedipus* and Tom McGrath's *Electra*), *Three Sisters* (2000) and *Thebans* (2003) (based on Sophocles' *Oedipus* and *Antigone* and Euripides' *Phoenician Women*) complement two more Molières. *Miseryguts* (2002), her Glaswegian *Le Misanthrope*, finds contemporary targets for her satirical wit; *Educating Agnes* (2008) with a Glaswegian of colour originally cast as heroine is based on *L'École des Femmes*. Harris's *Further than the Furthest Thing* (2000), while clearly based on the evacuation of Tristan da Cunha in 1961 and the difficulties for its people of resettling in England, explores issues of (post)colonialism, community cohesion and disruption – and specific community language in ways that echo and reflect the work of other playwrights based, like her, in devolutionary Scotland. She tends to write between English national and Scottish companies. Her RSC trilogy *Midwinter* (2004), *Solstice* (2005) and *Fall* (2008), clearly inspired by recent Balkan conflicts, counterpoints work like her 2006 NTS version of *Miss Julie*, set during the 1926 General Strike.

Although Tosg collapsed in 2007 and Suspect Culture wound itself up in 2009, its founders' feeling they had completed what they wished for it, there remains a post-1999 vitality about Scotland's theatrical life. A key element of this is the NTS, already mentioned in relation to Harris and Burke plays and founded in 2006. Several twentieth-century attempts failed to establish a Scottish national theatre (Agnew 2000): by 1970, the Scottish Arts Council thought a touring company might develop, perhaps merging with Edinburgh's Royal Lyceum Company; from 1980, the Scottish Theatre Company employed a touring model, seeking to be a proto-national company. After what were widely seen as years of underfunding, it collapsed in 1987, when the Advisory Council for the Arts in Scotland (AdCAS) published a national theatre working party report. Despite AdCAS and the efforts of campaign leader Donald Smith, little publicly seemed to happen till the Federation of Scottish Theatre, Scotland's professional companies' representative body, argued post-devolution for the current non-building based co-production-focused model. In fact, in 1996 a Royal Lyceum Board member, Councillor Moira Knox, hosted a lunch for Lord Lindsay, Scottish Office junior minister, who offered the joint chief executives, Kenny Ireland and Nikki Axford, an additional million pounds annually to make the Lyceum a building-based national theatre. Both turned this down, considering it politically inappropriate both nationally and theatrically (Brown 2009: 220). (This may have been part of John Major's attempts to fend off devolution, which include the awarding of Scottish [and Welsh] Arts Council independence in 1994, something the present author has called 'a national theatre to deny a national settlement' [Brown 2009: 220].) The building-based model would certainly have been divisive and old-fashioned. The post-devolution collaborative model is not only inclusive and forward-looking, but, quite consciously, avoids the capital-intensive dangers of buildings that not even the 1970 report or AdCAS evaded and which mark the national theatre models of England or France.

Michael Lynch has made the point vividly that Scotland has from the earliest times been a nation not unified by conquest, but formed by alliance and regional magnates working under a *primus inter pares* high king (Lynch 1991). Scotland perceives itself as part of a continuum diachronically, not only over the centuries since the old 'sang endit', but at least over two millennia. It is also a synchronic continuum, as this chapter has argued, for the range of theatre leading into and out of 1979–99. The NTS, with no single centre, its focus on co-producing with other Scottish companies, a *prima inter pares* of modern Scotland's dramatic magnates, marks new, progressive and visionary theatrical confidence. Its first production in February 2006 was famously not an establishment city-bound classic. It was *Home*, ten different new productions from Shetland to Dumfries, Stornoway to Aberdeen. Each adopted specific local/national approaches to that theme. Each launched the continuing process, one of 'Scotlands' rather than 'Scotland', 'events' rather than an 'event'. Scotland has a new, and still developing, constitutional settlement, explored and sustained by its theatre. Key to post-devolutionary Scottish theatre is that it remains, in the broadest sense, effective and dynamic politically as well as culturally.

Works cited

Agnew, D. (2000), *Contexts and Concepts of a Scottish National Theatre*, unpublished PhD thesis, Queen Margaret University.

Archibald, D. (2008), '"We're just big bullies" … Gregory Burke's *Black Watch*', *The Drouth*, No. 26 (Winter), pp. 8–13.

Beveridge, C., and Turnbull, R. (1989), *The Eclipse of Scottish Culture*, Edinburgh: Polygon.

Brown, I. (1984), 'Cultural Centrality and Dominance: The Creative Writer's View – Conversations with Scottish Poet/Playwrights', *Interface*, No. 3 (Summer), pp. 17–67; also now available on-line in *International Journal of Scottish Theatre and Screen*, vol. 4, no. 1 (2011) at http://journals.qmu.ac.uk/index.php/IJOSTS/article/view/118.

—— (2007), 'Staging the Nation: Multiplicity and Cultural Diversity in Contemporary Scottish Theatre' in Ian Brown et al. (eds.), *The Edinburgh History of Scottish Literature*, Edinburgh: Edinburgh University Press, pp. 283–194.

—— (2009), 'Entering the Twenty-first Century', in Ian Brown and Alan Riach (eds.), *The Edinburgh Companion to Twentieth-Century Scottish Literature*, Edinburgh: Edinburgh University Press, pp. 214–22.

Brown, I., and Nicholson, C. (2007), 'The Border Crossers and Reconfiguration of the Possible: Poet-Playwright-Novelists from the Mid-twentieth Century on', in Ian Brown et al. (eds.), *The Edinburgh History of Scottish Literature*, Edinburgh: Edinburgh University Press, pp. 262–272.

Brown, I., Clancy, T. O., Manning. S., and Pittock, M. (2007), *The Edinburgh History of Scottish Literature*, Edinburgh: Edinburgh University Press, pp. 262–272.

Corbett, J. (1999), *Written in the Language of the Scottish Nation: A History of Literary Translation into Scots*, Clevedon: Multilingual Matters.

Craig, C. (1996), *Out of History: Narrative Paradigms in Scottish and English Culture*, Edinburgh: Polygon.

Gifford, D. (2007), 'Breaking Boundaries: From Modern to Contemporary in Scottish Fiction' in Ian Brown et al. (eds.), *The Edinburgh History of Scottish Literature*, Edinburgh: Edinburgh University Press, pp. 237–252.

Lenz, K. (1996), 'Modern Scottish Drama: Snakes in Iceland – Drama in Scotland?', *Zeitschrift für Anglistik und Amerikanistik*, Vol. XLIV, no. 4, pp. 301–16.

—— (1999), *Die schottische Sprache im modernen Drama*, Universitätsverlag C. Winter: Heidelberg.

Lynch, M. (1991), *Scotland: A New History*, London: Century.

McClure, J. D. (1988), *Why Scots Matters*, Edinburgh: The Saltire Society.

—— (1991), 'Is Translation Naturalisation? Some Test Cases from Scots', in J. J. Simon and A. Sinner (eds.) *English Studies 3: Proceedings of the Third Conference on the Literature of Region and Nation, Part 1*, Luxembourg: Publications des Centre Universitaire de Luxembourg.

Macleod, M., and Watson, M. (2007), 'In the Shadow of the Bard: The Gaelic Short Story, Novel and Drama since the early Twentieth Century', in Ian Brown et al. (eds.), *The Edinburgh History of Scottish Literature*, Edinburgh: Edinburgh University Press, pp. 273–282.

Macwhirter, I. (2007), 'Eventful Times as SNP See Home', *The Sunday Herald*, 18 August.

Maxwell, D. (2000), http://www.benharrison.info/productions/decky.htm. Accessed 29 November 2009.

Sassi, C. (2009), 'The (B)order in Modern Scottish Literature', in Ian Brown and Alan Riach (eds.), *The Edinburgh Companion to Twentieth-Century Scottish Literature*, Edinburgh: Edinburgh University Press, pp. 145–155.

Chapter 3

Theatre and Performance in a Devolved Wales

Steve Blandford

For a stateless nation such as Wales the creation of national institutions is an almost inevitable part of the endless struggle to establish an identity, usually in the shadow of a much larger or more powerful neighbour. The way that such institutions are constituted, however, will determine whether or not they are monolithic pale imitations of the same thing that exists elsewhere within the larger state or whether they will offer a framework in which a constant process of, in Benedict Anderson's (1983) terms, imagining the nation can take place.

To those both inside and outside Wales it will then be of inescapably powerful symbolic value that Wales has chosen to create two national theatre institutions during the last decade. The first of these to be created was Theatr Genedlaethol Cymru launched in 2003, and the second was National Theatre Wales launched in 2008. As the two names suggest, the former operates in the Welsh language, the latter in English. The following chapter will not only explore the significance of the setting up of two companies, but also the often highly charged political significance of theatre in Wales, particularly in the period since 1997.

In the period since the establishment of the Wales Assembly Government in 1999 as part of the UK government's programme of devolution that began in 1997, theatre in Wales has been something of a political battleground. The relatively limited powers of the Assembly government (especially in the initial phase of devolution) inevitably gave areas such as cultural policy a particularly sharp focus. A theatre heavily dependent on state funding via the Arts Council of Wales was frequently on the front line of debate not just about theatre, but about the kind of new nation that was emerging.

In many ways it is possible to read this as very positive. The engagement of the Assembly government, the media in Wales and, to some extent, the public in debates about what kind of theatre the new nation should support through public subsidy could be seen as a welcome recognition of the role of the art form in the imagining of the new nation. Such recognition was also seen in the relatively prominent role played by theatre makers in public debate around the devolution referendum of 1997. Ed Thomas, one of the most successful writers for theatre, film and television to emerge from Wales in the late twentieth century, was a particularly prominent media commentator during the campaign for a 'Yes' vote in the referendum, and his words in a national newspaper around that time have become an oft-quoted mantra for those who saw the possibility of national reinvention in a devolved Wales:

Old Wales is dead. The Wales of stereotype, leeks, daffodils, look-you-now boyo rugby supporters singing Max Boyce songs in three-part harmony while phoning mam to tell her they'll be home for tea and Welsh cakes has gone [...] So where does it leave us? Free to make up, re-invent, redefine our own versions of Wales, all three million definitions if necessary, because the Wales I know is bilingual, multicultural, pro-European, messed up, screwed up and ludicrously represented in the British press [...] So old Wales is dead and new Wales is already a possibility, an eclectic self-defined Wales with attitude.

(Quoted in Roms 1998: 186)

For Thomas the writer of theatre, films and television, devolution offered impetus and new possibilities to those who felt Wales to be a place of possibility and, in turn, artists had the opportunity to contribute to the continuous reinvention of the country. In a way that was paralleled in Scotland with the involvement of writers such as David Greig in the Scottish devolution campaign, the creators of fictional narratives were seen as an integral part of the re-writing of the nation.

It would be wrong of course to imply in any way that this was a phenomenon that began with political devolution. Not only is the idea of a national theatre for Wales over a century old (see Jones 2007, for a detailed discussion), but the use of theatre and performance as a means of exploring national identity was a strong pre-occupation of artists in Wales well before the impetus for devolution had been given new momentum by the incoming Labour government in 1997.

At its best this pre-occupation took the form of a genuine search for what David Adams called, '[...] a new, vibrant and distinctive theatre tradition in Wales, one which is relevant and responsive to the perceptions, experience, aspirations and concerns of a minority culture and a small nation and which is more than just a pale reflection of English theatre convention' (1996: 5).

Such work in the 1980s and 1990s included internationally renowned theatre 'experiments' by companies such as Brith Gof, Moving Being and Volcano who many recognised as being better known internationally than they were in the UK. Though never confined by the exploration of Welsh identity it could reasonably be claimed that, particularly for Brith Gof, the idea of a separate Wales was a constant and recurring theme. However, as Jen Harvie explains, the theatrical exploration of such ideas in Brith Gof's work was never in the spirit of revealing a single 'authentic' sense of Welshness, but rather about the contested nature of the nation's identity from the beginning of its often turbulent history. Here Harvie discusses *Gododdin*, one of Brith Gof's key performances with respect to the company's significant contribution to ideas of Welsh identity and its relationship to an often mythologised past:

Gododdin remembered and constituted a strong and often positive narrative of Welsh identity as linguistically and culturally rich, loyal, creative, innovative, and brave, whether in the face of war, environmental onslaught or economic decline. It did not, however, present an entirely unified sense of national identity that might then be seen as fixed or, indeed, exclusive and xenophobic. McLucas [a key member of Brith Gof] argued, 'The idea of an authentic Welshness which speaks for the heartland is a myth'.

(Harvie 2005: 49–50)

Arguably it is the vein that Harvie identifies here in Brith Gof's work, but which was also prominent in a variety of other theatre artists, that was the saving grace of a culture frequently characterised by an intense pre-occupation with national identity. A pre-occupation that is often associated with small nations in particular kinds of relationships with larger, more powerful neighbours. By saving grace I mean a determination to identify complexity and constant evolution as the most important characteristics of a drama concerned with nations and national identity, rather than a search for spurious authenticity.

Many, not only in Wales, have wanted to go much further and argue for art in the pursuit of a post-national ideal, particularly in the light of some of the horrors committed in the name of nationalism in the last two decades. This very point was in fact at the heart of one of Brith Gof's later works, *Prydian: The Impossibility of Britishness* (1996). In the programme notes for *Prydian* the company expresses such a position very explicitly: 'After the break-up of former Yugoslavia can the idea of nation have any credibility when unspeakable acts were committed in its name?' (quoted in Roms 2004: 186). In fact, as Roms goes on to suggest, the work was less pessimistic about the idea of the nation than this sentence implies, but the idea of a post-national Wales is one that has received serious and sustained discussion in the period since devolution. As the historian Chris Williams puts it:

Discourses of nationality operate by 'othering', by identifying borders between 'us' and 'them'. Such reactive and essentialist binarisms erect psychological barriers between peoples, excite unnecessary antagonisms towards others, and render marginal or invisible those whose characteristics do not fit those of the imagined nation [...] They close frontiers both internally and externally. In Wales we would do well to avoid what Said called the 'rhetoric of blame' that often exists between imperial and newly independent states, and to refrain from indulging in an anachronistic burst of nation-building, just as the nation-state finally begins to recede from its central position on the world stage. A 'post-national' Wales is a more attractive prospect.

(Williams 2005: 16)

For the most part, whether or not they have engaged with the idea of the nation, the majority of significant Welsh theatre practitioners have avoided the advocacy of what Williams calls an 'anachronistic burst of nation building', and have instead exploited the ability of theatre to play out the inherent fluidity of ideas of national identity, particularly during times of political change. However the formation of national institutions such as theatres is never without controversy and we will return more specifically to this later in the chapter. Before that, it is worth briefly surveying some of the key engagements with the idea of the national that have been made outside the framework of institution building.

If, for Chris Williams, Welsh thinkers and artists had been given an opportunity to at least explore the utopian idea of the nation state there were also progressive thinkers who saw dangers in such a position, particularly with regard to Wales' historical legacy as part of Britain:

> Whilst the possibility of constructing human communities capable of cooperation and of maintaining a wealth of cultural diversity while eschewing nationhood may be an ideal worth working for, for contemporary Wales to give up its aspirations to nationhood surely would do little to further that cause. The post-nation people of Wales could not float in limbo in a world otherwise inhabited by nationals without being recatergorised: we would all, willy-nilly, be categorised by others if not by ourselves, as 'British', as unproblematic members of the British nation-state. And in today's Britain, the default position for those who identify, or are identified, as British only, with no qualifiers, remains an unexamined English cultural identity.
>
> (Aaron 2005: 155)

Written in the period immediately following the Iraq war and at a time when a newly strengthened Anglo-American alliance was finding itself increasingly isolated in the world, Jane Aaron's idea of newly defined Wales was persuasive and it is this position rather than the more radical post-national ideal that has tended to prevail in the making of theatre and performance in the period since devolution.

Engagement with the national by Welsh makers of theatre and performance in this period has, fortunately, taken endlessly different forms and it is worth a brief survey of this broad spectrum before returning again to the specific question of national theatres.

Perhaps understandably, the start of this decade saw a number of high profile, very direct attempts to situate any sense of a new, confident Wales (the now much-derided idea of 'Cool Cymru') firmly within the realities of post-industrialisation. Work such as Patrick Jones' *Everything Must Go* (1999), Helen Griffin's *Flesh and Blood* (2000) and Ian Rowlands' *New South Wales* (1999) all variously used their characters' sense of something new emerging in Wales to sound warnings about the new country while simultaneously acknowledging a new excitement and the potential that this had for effecting social, economic and cultural change.

Everything Must Go attracted particular attention because its author, Patrick Jones, is the brother of Nicky Wire of The Manic Street Preachers and one of a clutch of internationally successful Welsh popular musicians that were the main focus of the unwelcome 'Cool Cymru' label that circulated widely in the press in the late 1990s (see Blandford 2000). Produced by Cardiff's Sherman Theatre Company, *Everything Must Go*, later transferred for a short run at The Tricycle Theatre, Kilburn, and, in common with many cultural events from Wales before it, was much better received by critics from London than many in Wales (though it was very popular with younger Welsh audiences).

Barely a year after the opening of the Welsh Assembly, Jones' play offered a dystopian vision of a Wales as a source of cheap labour, dominated by call centres and factories making electronic products for Japanese and Korean companies. Partly through the use of the Manic Street Preachers' music and a highly charged melodramatic plot, the play played to large audiences in Cardiff and London, many of them not regular theatre goers. As some reviewers at the time suggested, the play was somewhat out of step with what Aleks Sierz later labelled 'In-Yer-Face Theatre' (2001) in that it was unafraid of both political and emotional directness:

Unlike the Trainspottings and Shopping and F***ings, the play is an astute portrayal of working-class disaffection that does not shy away from presenting articulate characters and the politics not just of today but of 50 years ago. There is no space here for post-modern disdain towards any cultural references that predate Bagpuss; here are two drug-fuelled monologues angled towards Aneurin Bevan and five dedicated to the great mid-century ills he fought against: Want, Disease, Ignorance, Idleness and Squalor.

(Judah 2000)

Similarly Helen Griffin's *Flesh and Blood* (2000), though perhaps less politically direct than *Everything Must Go*, asked severe questions about the certainties of any putative, postcolonial Welsh dawn. As one reviewer put it:

Hidden behind the façade of Cool Cymru lies a Wales ravaged by unemployment, racial tensions and fear for the future. Helen Griffin's first full-length play wrestles with all these ideas in this bittersweet black comedy, using one Swansea family as a metaphor for a nation.

(Watts 2000)

If Griffin and Jones could both claim to have produced engaging, populist work that provided dissenting voices amid the epidemic of post-devolutionary optimism, they both also attracted strong criticism for what some saw as unsophisticated naturalism on the one hand and raw political sloganising on the other. Viewed as direct opposition to this kind of trend was the work of one of the most celebrated of contemporary Welsh writers, Ian Rowlands. David Adams' reading of Rowlands is at the heart of what sometimes seems a somewhat desperate attempt to define Welsh theatre by its simple opposition to a mythical 'English' version; '[...] he [Rowlands] also abrogates and appropriates theatrical convention by subverting the traditional naturalism of English theatre' (Adams 1999: 252).

Adams' view of Rowlands has the potential to resonate throughout this volume in its anxiety to pin down and assert postcolonial difference in the artists of small or emergent nations. To suggest that the rejection of realist/naturalist forms is in itself an act of postcolonial resistance is to misunderstand the complexity and diversity of both English and Welsh theatrical culture. Rowlands' theatrical struggles in search of intelligent ways to think about Welsh identity risk being undone by such simplicities, especially as they submerge true complexity beneath the weight of an outmoded English/Welsh binary opposition. In fact, in Rowlands' more direct homage to the moment of devolution itself, we hear one of his characters implicitly criticise the desirability of such a way of thinking, 'The only thing the Welsh can agree upon is what they're not – not English' (Rowlands, 1999, unpublished).

More sophisticated academic attempts to examine the distinctiveness of a Welsh performance tradition have, however, been made and in 2004 the UK Journal *Studies in Theatre and Performance* published a 'Welsh Theatre Special Issue' with its editorial proclaiming, 'This is no doubt (sic) that this issue of *Studies in Theatre and Performance* deals with a distinct 'case-study': the national arena of Wales' (Harper 2004: 149).

Interestingly and slightly curiously, the edition avoids very much direct engagement with what then becomes the elephant in the room, namely the arrival of a Welsh-language national theatre and the consequent hotting-up of the debate as to whether this now meant that there must be a parallel development working in the English language. Though many of the articles are more explicit about their opposition to the idea of 'national theatres', another editorial's argues that '[a]ny discussion of the need for the creation of any national theatre for Wales is redundant, because the politicians see it as part of the nation-building project' (Ros 2004a: 147). The stated will of the politicians should not of course be seen as an obstacle to debate among academics, of course, but it is perhaps understandable that serious commentators on theatre in Wales should seek to escape the prison of endless debates about the necessity of national institutions. The authors of the different articles then take oblique approaches, trying to open up what they see as theatrical spaces unique to Wales and in so doing to identify elements of the national in the theatre and performance traditions of the country and to cast doubt on the validity of debates about national theatres in the more conventional sense.

In some of the essays there are powerful arguments made for the avoidance of 'conventional theatre' (Ros 2004a: 147) at the heart of any really imaginative plans for the future of theatre and performance in the devolved Welsh nation. Ceri Sherlock's essay, while essentially true to its resonant final remarks – 'There is no conclusion, only process' (Sherlock 2004: 160) – does also come close to asserting an identity for theatre and performance in Wales that excludes a mainstream 'English' tradition of writer-led theatre:

That Wales has vital traditions in physical theatre, community theatre, and young people's theatre that predicate their work on experiments with the relationship between audience and performer, word text and physical (body/movement) text is a matter of immense pride. This is where our tradition lies – if we feel the need to construct one. Its direct lineage is clearly 'the performative'. Here we have artists who engage with their art forms *and* their audiences. This is the modest, silent and fruitful mainstream of Welsh theatre seen in a variety of venues and spaces in Crymych, Caernafon, Felinfach, Aberdare, Abergwesyn, in Aberystwyth, Wrexham and Llanelli.

(Sherlock 2004: 156)

For those unfamiliar with Wales, the point of the place names is to emphasise the embrace of the margins and to suggest a democratising principle that is outside the understanding of what Sherlock views as the middle-class, middle-brow of 'conventional theatre'. This sense of the place of alternative theatrical and performance traditions in Welsh life is addressed as a more specifically linguistic question by Nic Ros:

> One of the great challenges for any aspect of the development of the twenty-first-century Wales is the need to simultaneously address monoglots and bilinguals without homogenisation. While some cultural forms such as music can transcend linguistic barriers, the problem for text-based theatre is obvious. In experimental performance, the work of Brith Gof and Eddie Ladd engages with the past and future of Wales's culture without the need to constantly quantify and justify their use of the two languages.
>
> (2004b: 218)

Using the postcolonial frame of reference that became common (though not uncontroversially so) after devolution, Ros discusses the work of Guillermo Gomez-Peña and his performances that engage with the experiences of Mexicans and Chicanos on the US-Mexico border. As Ros says, Gomez-Peña's work 'appeals for tolerance' from somewhere that is more sharply focused and economically divisive than Wales, but which has important lessons for those involved in cultural practice in a Welsh context:

> It is time to face the facts: Anglos won't go back to Europe, and Mexicans and Latinos (legal or illegal) won't go back to Latin America. We are all here to stay. For better or worse, our destinies and aspirations are in one another's hands. For me the only solution lies in a paradigm shift: the recognition that we are all the protagonists in the creation of a new cultural topography and a new social order, one in which we are all "others", and we need the "others" to exist. Hybridity is no longer up for discussion. It is a demographic, racial, social and cultural fact.
>
> (Gomez-Peña 1995: 34)

Of course acceptance of a hybrid culture is one thing and a creative response is another. Since the special edition of *Studies in Theatre and Performance,* Theatr Genedlaethol Cymru (the Welsh-language national theatre of Wales) has been joined by National Theatre Wales. Despite the misgivings and objections (some of them in the special edition), the Welsh Assembly Government agreed to set aside special funding for the new theatre (to be administered by the Welsh Arts Council, who deserve great credit for convincing the devolved government of the case for a national theatre) for three years in the first instance and starting in 2008. This section of the chapter will conclude with some comment on that process and what the early work of National Theatre Wales suggests about its current and future role in the life of Wales and the international theatre community.

To begin with the most obvious, National Theatre Wales drew heavily on the inspiration of the National Theatre of Scotland which was set up in 2006. While there were differences that took account of the different contexts several of the important features were the same: no 'home' theatre building, a company light on permanent staff and seeking to work, at least part of the time, with partners either in existing organisations or as freelance proposers of projects on different scales. In both cases then great care was taken to avoid the charge of a monolithic 'trophy' organisation with a large expensive base inaccessible to large parts of the population that it had been set up to serve.

Key differences between both the Welsh and Scottish political devolution settlements and, more importantly in this case, the respective theatrical cultures and infrastructures in each nation, meant that there were necessary key differences between the way that National Theatre Wales and the National Theatre of Scotland were set up. The most obvious of these was the lack in Wales of the range of producing theatres that Scotland had, set alongside the much smaller population of Wales and the consequent lack of the same number of large urban centres of population. More contentiously it has long been argued that Wales has not had anything like the same strong playwriting tradition as Scotland with a consequently less-developed contemporary writing scene that any new national theatre could take immediate advantage of. Finally, of course, the National Theatre of Scotland while taking account of the general cultural diversity of contemporary Scotland did not have to take account of another established national theatre working through Gaelic (or any other language), nor indeed the very different linguistic context to be found in a bilingual Wales in general.

For many of the above reasons, the creation of National Theatre Wales was, to an extent, treated as something of a curiosity in sections of the UK press: 'With its stronger poetic tradition and bilingualism, Wales has not been fertile ground for theatre, which is what makes the birth of a new national theatre in English – a Welsh-language one already exists – so dramatic' (Moss, 2010). While the article is not unsympathetic, its overall tone is of detached amusement at the various obstacles that a national theatre faces in a small nation such as Wales:

> In some ways, necessity has been the mother of artistic invention. There wasn't enough money to build a new theatre, and in any case where would you put it? Someone would be irked: as Boyd Clack, who stars in *A Good Night Out* [National Theatre Wales' opening production], remarks, the Welsh are susceptible to jealousy. Better, and certainly cheaper, to establish a peripatetic company that takes theatre to people all over Wales. That, anyway, is the hope – although, as Clack also points out, the people already have their own theatre: fighting, drinking, sport and television.
>
> (Moss 2010)

Later on in the piece there is also oblique reference to the divisiveness of language issues as a 'Welsh language publication' is quoted as saying that the opening piece is 'provincial'. To an extent of course all this is not only inevitable, but healthy. It can be read as a sign of a culture ready to be open about its divisions and engaged enough in its cultural institutions for them to be contested territory. Certainly this piece and many others allows time and space for the company to express its inclusive values and determination to engage with the 'idea' of Wales as in this explanation by the artistic director John E. McGrath:

> 'We're called the National Theatre Wales, so we're asking: what does that mean?' says McGrath. 'If you're touring a production, in a way you have to come up with one unified thing and take it on tour, whereas by working in 12 different places you can ask that question afresh each time you make a piece of work. You can look at a nation through history, through identity, but really we thought what a nation is is a place – so let's explore what place means.'
>
> (Moss 2010)

McGrath's '12 different places' refers to the company's launch year which premiered 12 pieces of work in 12 locations across Wales in 2010-11. This hugely ambitious project which involved working with numerous partnerships and individual artists was a powerful political gesture as well as a fascinating aesthetic challenge. The locations ranged from traditional theatre spaces in cities to games-based work on beaches, a contemporary reworking of Aeschyclus' *The Persians* on the huge army firing ranges of the Brecon Beacons National Park and, most spectacularly of all, the staging of *The Passion* in Port Talbot with text by Owen Sheers. The latter was a collaboration between National Theatre Wales, WildWorks (an internationally renowned company, specialising in large-scale site specific work) and the Port Talbot-born actor Michael Sheen whose commitment to the production was widely seen as testimony to the strength of the vision for a national theatre that the company has sought to establish in its first year of existence. Even more significantly perhaps is that, at the conclusion of its three days over Easter 2011, the production was not only seen by an estimated 12000 people but also included over 1000 participants from the Port Talbot area. As many critics recognised, this was theatre that genuinely looked beyond its traditional boundaries and which successfully married a deep commitment to the communities to which it belongs with an excellence that brought international acclaim.

Perhaps most of all, the launch year was a challenge to those who opposed the idea of national theatre for Wales in any form because, in postcolonial terms they feared the subaltern mentality. For such critics the very idea of a national theatre betrayed the unique performance culture of Wales in favour of a something adopted from the dominant European imperial model. What National Theatre Wales was attempting to do (and as I write the launch year is only just coming to a conclusion), and what the National Theatre of Scotland has been attempting in slightly different ways, is to reinvent and repossess the very idea of a national theatre and, to some extent, the very idea of the nation.

If the core of this re-invention of a national theatre is the decentralisation of the production base, then in small ways National Theatre Wales has sought to take this a step further. Part of this is about reaching out to new audiences, but also in a geographically dispersed country the company's inventive and inclusive online presence is a practical as well as a philosophical statement. From its inception National Theatre Wales's creation of a community has had online social networks at its heart. It deliberately delayed the launch of any official website until well after its own social network had grown to a credible size in order that its followers would feel part of the original public face of the company's work. Open groups within the social network of actors, writers, directors and designers are National Theatre Wales' preferred means of communication not just with its audiences, but with its potential collaborators and of course the network is alive with blogs, posts and frequently lively debate. It is a deliberately slightly anarchic way to 'meet' a national institution, but it marks out National Theatre Wales as genuinely distinctive.

While this chapter can hardly be the final word on a venture very much in its infancy, the importance to the Welsh nation of National Theatre Wales has become widely recognised both inside and outside the country. The liberal arts establishment in the rest of the UK has pronounced itself quite excited and in some cases very much convinced about the role of the company in the continuing project to establish the idea of a Britain that has a devolved (some even use the word federal) structure:

> Diversity – thematic, stylistic and geographical – is the name of the game for National Theatre Wales. And one of their achievements is to have raised our consciousness about their country. A young Welsh critic asked me how I, as someone based in London, reacted to the theatre company. I said, truthfully, that it had opened my somewhat blinkered metropolitan eyes. In the past, I've paid random visits to Cardiff for Welsh National Opera and to north Wales to see the work of Teatr Clwyd. Now, I'm belatedly waking up to the rich potential of Welsh theatre and the variety of the land itself. Driving to Blackwood to see the company's opening show, *A Good Night Out in the Valleys,* I saw for the first time a Wales I knew only from books, movies and TV programmes.
>
> (Billington 2010)

Later in the same piece Billington uses the term 'immersive' to describe the approach of some elements of National Theatre Wales' first year and cross-refers to the work of the English theatre company Punchdrunk only to own up to the fact that such work has been common in Wales for many years. Whether the term immersive is quite the right one is probably not worth debating, but perhaps Billington's remarks do sum up well the dual function of the reinvention of the idea of national theatre in small nations such as Wales and Scotland. Not only are they engaged in the continuous reimagination of the national present they also have the capacity to encourage reappraisal of the cultural past. For those who saw Wales as a place that had little or no theatrical tradition and needed a national theatre to invent one are perhaps discovering that National Theatre Wales is about connecting the world to an undiscovered past as well as inventing a future that embraces the possibilities in new form of social connection.

Before concluding this chapter with some analysis of the progress of work in the Welsh language, it is worth reflecting for a moment on the role of the playwright in

English-speaking Welsh theatre culture. It has become almost axiomatic both inside and outside Wales to assert that the bilingual nature of Welsh public life both works against the idea of the writer and encourages forms of performance that are visual and less reliant on text. Jen Harvie quotes Mike Pearson, founder of Brith Gof as seeing this as an advantage, and one that encouraged the rich traditions of visual, physical and site-specific theatre and performance that has flourished in Wales during the last three decades:

> 'With no mainstream tradition defining what theatre ought to look like, and with no national theatre prescribing an orthodoxy of theatrical convention, with no great wealth of playwriting,' Pearson argued, 'then theatre in Wales still has options. It has the chance to address different subject-matters, using different means, in spaces other than the silent and darkened halls of theatre auditoria'.
>
> (Harvie 2005: 46)

While this position is entirely understandable and acknowledges the extraordinary tradition that Pearson and others helped to foster in Wales, it tends to exclude the emergence of writers in a way that almost suggests that this kind of work could be antithetical to a progressive vision of Welsh theatre. National Theatre Wales has the potential to foster the idea that new writing for the theatre can be a genuinely significant part of the theatre and performance landscape in Wales and its commissioning both of new work for its first year of production and of writers developing work for the future suggests that this is part of its agenda.

One of National Theatre Wales' first commissioned writers is Gary Owen who, since devolution, has produced a body of work that makes him probably the most significant playwright to have emerged in Wales in that time and one whose work demonstrates both a commitment to tell stories of the place where he lives and works, but who is not confined by traditional ideas of the nation and identity. Via productions with the National Theatre (London) and Paines Plough, then the leading UK-based new writing company, Owen's writer's journey has taken him back to Wales and to Welsh-based commissions, something he associates directly with his view of the role of the writer in contemporary public life. Here he describes the impetus behind his decision to accept a commission from National Theatre Wales to write a play that reflected on the so-called 'Bridgend suicides', the often-distorted (by the UK national press) number of young people living in the County Borough of Bridgend in South Wales that took their own lives during the middle years of the last decade:

> Why I'm doing this now is that in addition to being a writer from Bridgend, I believe publicly-funded theatre has a role in democracy. I don't think you can shirk from taking on the big topics and what's important is that this work will happen in Bridgend with and for the people of Bridgend.
>
> (Owen 2010)

If Owen's very clear and welcome statement of both writers' and publicly funded theatre's role in democracy has a general truth and energising potential for the contemporary writer, then it can be argued that it is doubly true for small nations such as Wales. Owen's work as a writer from the early *Crazy Gary's Mobile Disco* (2001) has sought to engage with the society and culture from which he came, but also to avoid the conventional pitfalls of sloganising about the idea of the nation and national identity. If there is a link between them all, they tend to be plays about the marginalised within a culture that has often defined itself through its own marginality. It is therefore of some significance that one of the ways in which a new national theatrical culture is being established in Wales is through a re-thinking of some of the old polarities and in so doing re-thinking the idea that a bilingual culture is inimical to the idea of playwright.

To conclude this chapter on theatre and performance in Wales, I want to turn now to theatre and performance in the Welsh language since devolution. To begin with of course it is important to recognise that this is a false and somewhat distorted division. A number of the significant Welsh companies of recent years have frequently used both Welsh and English in their work. This is especially true of performances dominated by the physical and visual, but there are also examples of writers producing bilingual work including Gary Owen, whose 2009 work *Amgen* will be discussed briefly below. However, it is also clear that the establishment of Theatr Genedlaethol Cymru and the existence of companies with strong international profiles such as Theatr Bara Caws indicates both an appetite and political will for theatre predominantly in the Welsh language.

That it was politically possible to establish a national theatre institution working exclusively in Welsh some five years before its English-language counterpart is not without significance, but neither should that significance be overplayed. It should, for example, be seen in the context of the existence of significant public funding for theatre in English and the steady growth of Welsh-language education in areas of south Wales where Welsh had previously been in a long steady decline. Nevertheless, allocation of new funding to establish Theatr Genedlaethol, although modest, was a clear statement of priorities by the Welsh Assembly Government and one welcomed as a new opening up of possibilities for those working in Welsh in the devolved nation. At the time of writing, some seven years on from the creation of a the company, there remains goodwill in Wales towards the idea of a national theatre working in Welsh (especially as there is now an English-language counterpart), but also a lingering sense of disappointment at what the company has been able to achieve. Ian Rowlands, in a lecture to the Welsh literature agency Academi spoke for many when he said:

For me, Theatr Genedlaethol Cymru (the National Theatre of Wales), or rather Theatr Genedlaethol y Cymry (the National Theatre of the Welsh) – one must define clearly – has proved, thus far, a missed opportunity – a purveyor of miss-truths! I expected truth, quality and vision from the new company – and expected in vain. Time after time I have been disappointed by the company's work, and yet I have faith in the basic nature of the ideal [...] there was, and still is, very little co-operation in the Welsh-language theatre. Theatre in this country is usually created by dictatorship, there is very little consideration of the greater good; very little shared aspiration.

My disappointment with the current company stems from the fact that it is a continuation of the old insular and parochial way. I believe very strongly in the purpose and role of a National Theatre in a civilised nation; a theatre that stages the individual's truths in a community of communities. For any nation to support a national company which does not reflect the aspirations of the country is wasteful.

(Rowlands 2007)

Essentially Rowlands argument hinges on quality and ambition, or rather the lack of it in the work of the company, and what he sees as a reliance on an insular nationalism for its own sake. For Rowlands it would be infinitely preferable to have just one national theatre that operated not only in English and Welsh even, but one that recognised the true diversity of a modern Wales, linguistic and otherwise:

Had Theatr Genedlaethol y Cymry the vision, I suggest it could venture on a revolutionary course; artistically and socially. Were the board of Theatr Genedlaethol y Cymry to vote to refuse its million a year, and to insist the money allocated to the Welsh-language theatre be an integral part of the integrated provision of the proposed national theatre, that could ensure an equal future for the Welsh-language expression alongside the English-language expression. It is too easy to isolate the Welsh language – the establishment has long known how to do so. Strength lies in unity – together we succeed!

Mrs Jones Llanrug and her peers are a dying breed. The future is not theirs. The older generation deserve our respect, but the future belongs to the young and they have different values; new expectations of their theatre.

They are confident of their identity, reaching out and insisting on being part of the wider community. They crave to build bridges and to communicate. Wales today is the Wales of the young at heart, and theatre should reflect that. That is the role of theatre, to mirror its audience, to be a stage for its ambition; to offer its hopes a voice, to insist on a better world. Alun Lewis wrote, 'The world is much larger than just England, isn't it? I'll never be just English or Welsh again.' For too long, the world has been black and white for the Welsh. It's high time the nation saw the whole spectrum. One theatre, several voices. One voice, several languages [...]

(Rowlands 2007)

It is not my intention here to fully debate Rowlands' indictment of Theatr Genedlaethol Cymru's output to date, but there is a clear sense within Wales that its staple touring diet of classics translated into Welsh and Welsh-language classics interspersed with the odd new commission has failed to establish a reputation that sits comfortably with the idea of 'national' theatres.

There are exceptions of course, and the revival of Saunders Lewis's *Esther* in 2006 brought the actor Daniel Evans back to Wales to direct. In contrast to much of the company's work, the design of the show was stark and almost oppressive in keeping with the play's themes of great sacrifice and suffering. While the staging of Lewis's work would clearly be a predictable part of the company's repertoire, the production was of the highest quality and the enticing of an actor/director of Evans' stature back to Wales to direct after London and Broadway successes is very much part of the reason for creating such a strong institution working in Welsh.

Equally, the 2008 production of a new play, *Iesu!* by Aled Jones Williams, performed one of the principal functions of all theatre which is to incite debate and controversy. Staged in Cardiff during the National Eisteddfod, the play has Jesus as a female figure with the design creating unmistakable echoes of the photos from Guantanamo and Abu Ghraib. In the scene most frequently reported on by reviewers, Jesus is raped by soldiers as Pilate looks on. At key moments quotations from George W. Bush and Donald Rumsfeld appear on a screen. To add further to the cocktail, the playwright earns his living as a Church in Wales minister in Porthmadog.

For those who saw it, what was most significant about *Iesu!* in the life of Theatr Genedlaethol was the attempt to create main-stage theatre in Welsh that spoke firmly to the contemporary context outside the confines of the Welsh experience. In other words theatre that demonstrated that the Welsh language remained a real vehicle through which its speakers could engage fully with the world and that was capable of enriching modern life and experience. Later in Ian Rowlands' critical lecture quoted from above he says:

> I dream of theatre of a high standard in Wales; theatre relevant to the whole nation and to the world beyond the confines of our historical prejudices; the narrowness, which chokes the development not only of the art form, but also of our nation.
>
> (Rowlands 2007)

In *Iesu!* there is a case for saying that Theatr Genedlaethol Cymru demonstrated the potential for a national theatre in the Welsh language to fulfill Rowlands' dream, but that it has yet to do this with any level of consistency.

There is, of course, more to Welsh-language theatre than the national institution created to further its cause. Wales has a funded network of companies providing theatre for young people in both English and Welsh that is internationally almost unique (though constantly vulnerable to the vagaries of funding cuts as we enter the so-called age of austerity). This includes Theatr Iolo, Gwent Theatre, Theatr Na N'Og, Arad Goch, Fran Wen and Theatr Powys, many of whom commission new work from writers in both languages. Sera Moore Williams, one of the most significant contemporary

Welsh-language playwrights worked for many years at Arad Goch consistently producing work that challenges outsiders' views of the rural heartlands of the north and west of Wales. A number of the projects that Arad Goch created have involved young people from challenging backgrounds, and Sera Moore Williams observations on this kind of work open up fascinating questions about language, identity and theatre in Wales. Discussing one project in rural Ceredigion, Williams says:

> Although the language of the projects is always predominantly English, the actors who work with us are bilingual, and we actively encourage anyone who can to speak Welsh to us. Most of the young people initially deny that they can speak Welsh, possibly because their main experience of the language has been at school, and school for the most part has very negative connotations for most of them. It's been a joy, and possibly a measure of the success of the work, to see the language being reclaimed as something that for the first time for them probably has some status attached to it. During each project people who have been extremely reluctant to speak Welsh have begun to relish their ability to speak a word here or a sentence there.
>
> (Williams 2004: 94)

Not only does this account actively question the familiar picture of north and west Wales as relatively harmonious havens dominated by farming and tourism, it also reveals much about the relationship between the Welsh language's struggle for survival and an active, vibrant theatre and performance scene that uses it as part of a meaningful contemporary culture that is embedded in the lives of young people.

Most recently, a small but increasingly significant body of work has begun to appear in which younger contemporary writers have made the active choice to express themselves bilingually. For many, this is a highly significant step and a pointer to a progressive vision of Wales's linguistic and artistic future. Gary Owen's *Amgen/Broken* (2009) was an attempt to explore the writer's own experiences of depression as a young man, but also to explore the potential of bilingual theatre to communicate with audiences that may or may not be able to use both languages.

Part of the point of *Amgen/Broken* is that it is a fundamentally different experience depending on whether you speak one or both of the languages. To an extent, this becomes a play about the fundamental nature of art as we refract the play through our own experiences and frames of reference. However, the choices made by Owen suggest something else. The play involves two characters: Gary who speaks in English and Gareth who speaks in Welsh. Gary's version of the world and the way that he presents himself is more controlled and ordered, whereas Gareth is chaotic and more erratic. Growing up as he did with a rudimentary form of bilingualism, but with English as his dominant language, Owen seems to be writing about the struggle with linguistic identity experienced by all young people in Wales, but perhaps most of all in the urban south of the country, furthest from the Welsh-speaking 'heartlands' and with a heritage formed most obviously through struggles of class and labour politics.

There is no sense of rejecting the Welsh language, but rather of struggling to make it fit into an already complex set of conflicted identities.

Finally, it is worth considering a recent bilingual production that had made arguably the most determined attempt to date to reach audiences beyond those that speak Welsh. Dafydd James' *Llywth* (2010), which translates as 'Tribe', is not only bilingual, but also uses a heavy Welsh/English dialect from south Wales, sometimes referred to as Wenglish. The performances also used surtitles in a further attempt to open up the work to a wider audience, something which resulted in a London fringe run, almost unheard of for a production that used a significant amount of Welsh.

Llywth is fundamentally about identity in the widest sense as it concerns a group of gay men on a night out in Cardiff when Wales have lost an international rugby match. The collisions of different ways of being Welsh are at the heart of the drama as the complications of being English-speaking, Welsh-speaking, bilingual, gay, straight or bisexual are played out against the backdrop of the fundamentals of an older, more straightforwardly masculine Wales – international rugby night in Cardiff. This is not, however, a sober meditation of identity, in fact it is a celebration of the hedonism of Cardiff's current nightlife, both gay and straight and is often very funny.

Through *Llywth* it is possible to glimpse an optimistic future for theatre and performance in Wales, a place that has struggled to emerge as a nation at all and which struggles with its own internal divisions and sense of its future. Here is a play that does not attempt to elide the divisions and complications inherent in what it means to be Welsh in the twenty-first century, but rather celebrates them as signs of life and vibrancy. As the generations who have experienced a basic bilingualism in their schooling grow up, as the generations who take political devolution and 'nationhood' for granted become adults, can we hope for a greater acceptance of hybridity in art forms including, at times, an intermingling of the languages of Wales?

Of course, theatre and performance makers need also to think beyond Welsh and English and consider the multiple linguistic and cultural identities that exist on the streets of Welsh towns and cities. They need to find creative ways to ask what it means to feel Welsh and Pakistani, Welsh and Somali, or Polish and particularly fond of Llanelli and a supporter of the Scarlets (rugby team). In going some way down this road and in turn mixing questions of national identity with ideas of sexuality and gender, *Llywth* becomes the kind of work through which a small nation can enjoy its own complexity, its own 'imagined communities', while also reaching out and telling its own stories to a wider world.

Such a brief discussion inevitably leaves out so much. The ever-inventive performance work of Eddie Ladd, Sean Tuan John and Marc Rees, the pioneering work in communities of Hijinx, a tiny company placed at the gleaming heart of Welsh cultural life through its home in the Wales Millenium Centre alongside Welsh National Opera, and playwrights emerging (sometimes remerging) in both languages, energised by the new opportunities of a National Theatre that seeks to engage with its artists on all levels. And yet, at the very moment of writing, a new era of cuts in government spending threatens us all. Considering the vibrancy and sheer hard work of the current scene and its sense of engagement with public life, it feels impossible that it can all disappear, though the scale of the cuts being proposed in a number of the Western European democracies has not been seen since the 1930s. It is a time of huge uncertainty. Perhaps though, we can finish with the hope that, if anywhere, it is in the small nations like Wales, where artists and politicians are in closest touch and where dialogue feels at least possible, that a strong theatre and performance culture, a potential source of democratic engagement and questioning, can survive.

Works cited

Aaron, J. (2005), 'Bardic Anti-colonialism' in Chris Williams and Jane Aaron (eds.) *Postcolonial Wales*, Cardiff: University of Wales Press.

Adams, D. (1996), *Stage Welsh*, Llandysul: Gomer.

—— (1999), 'Retrospective' in Ian Rowlands (ed.), *A Trilogy of Appropriation*, Cardiff: Parthian.

Anderson, B. (1983), *Imagined Communities: Reflections on the Origins and Spread of Nationalism*, London: Verso.

Billington, M. (2010), 'National Theatre Wales puts Cymru centre-stage', *The Guardian,* Theatre Blog, 1 June. Accessed June 2010.

Blandford, S. (2000), 'Aspects of the Live and Recorded Arts in Contemporary Wales', in David Dunkerley and Andrew Thompson (eds.), *Wales Today*, Cardiff: University of Wales Press, pp. 111–126.

Gomez-Peña, G. (1995), 'Border Art', in Richard Drain (ed.), *Twentieth Century Theatre: A Sourcebook*, London: Routledge.

Harper, G. (2004), 'Editorial: Performing Knowing', *Studies in Theatre and Performance*, 24: 3, p. 149.

Harvie, J. (2005), *Staging the UK*, Manchester: Manchester University Press.

Jones, A. (2007), *National Theatres in Context: France, Germany, England and Wales*, Cardiff: University of Wales Press.

Judah, H. (2000), '*Everything Must Go*', *The Times*, 15 May, http://www.theatre-wales.co.uk/plays/review_archive.asp?playname=Everything%20Must%20Go&company=Sherman%20Theatre%20Company. Accessed May 2010.

Moss, S. (2010), "National Theatre Wales' Roving Revolution', *The Guardian*, 1 March, http://www.guardian.co.uk/stage/2010/mar/01/national-theatre-wales. Accessed June 2010.

Owen, G. (2010), 'Gary Owen, Playwright', http://nationaltheatrewales.org/whatson/performance/ntw07#garyowenplaywright. Accessed July 2010.

Roms, H. (1998), 'Edward Thomas: A Profile', in Walford Davies H. (ed.), *State of Play: 4 Playwrights of Wales*, Llandysul: Gomer.

—— (2004), 'Performing *Polis*: theatre, nationess and civic identity in post-devolution Wales', *Studies in Theatre & Performance*, 24: 3, pp. 177–192.

Ros, N. (2004a), 'Editorial: Performance in Post-referendum Wales', *Studies in Theatre and Performance*, 24:3, pp. 147–148.

———— (2004b), 'Croesi'r llinell/Crossing the Line: Bilingualism in Post-referendum Welsh Theatre', *Studies in Theatre and Performance*, 24:3, pp. 205–219.

Rowlands, I. (1999), *New South Wales*, unpublished stage play.

———— (2007), Lecture to Academi Literary Lunch, Portmeirion, 30 September, http://www.academi.org/lectures/i/131389/. Accessed July 2010.

Sherlock, C. (2004), 'The Performative: Body – Text – Context and the Construction of a Tradition', *Studies in Theatre and Performance*, 24: 3, pp. 151–161.

Watts, R. (2000), *'Flesh and Blood'*, http://www.theatre-wales.co.uk/plays/review_archive.asp?playname=Flesh%20and%20Blood&company=Sherman%20Theatre%20Company. Accessed May 2010.

Williams, C. (2005), 'Problematising Wales: An Exploration in Historiography and Postcoloniality' in Chris Williams and Jane Aaron (eds.), *Postcolonial Wales*, Cardiff: University of Wales Press.

Williams, S. M. (2004), 'My Problem Sometimes', *New Welsh Review* (December), pp. 92–95.

Chapter 4

Contemporary Catalan Theatre and Identity: The Haunted Mirrors of Catalan Directors' Shakespeares

Helena Buffery

Sigui com sigui, el cos de la cultura catalana només pot créixer si pot accedir al mercat, si pot competir en la pista on els altres cossos normals practiquen la cursa d'obstacles. En un context mundial en què la cultura ha esdevingut una mercaderia, i en un context local en què la indústria cultural espanyola colonitza el mercat català, l'única possibilitat de supervivència de la cultura catalana és l'adopció d'estratègies que li permetin competir en els mateixos termes.[1]

(Fernàndez 2008: 40)

In his seminal study of the Catalan cultural field since 1976, Josep-Anton Fernàndez (2008) diagnoses the considerable malaise over questions of literary value, the relationship between language and culture and the marketability of Catalan cultural products, as a symptom of a crisis caused both by Catalonia's recent – and continuing – history of political and cultural subordination, and by the wider global crisis associated with postmodernity. His rigorous analysis of the causes and manifestations of this crisis are particularly sensitive to the implications of globalisation for small and, especially, stateless nations, which tend to have more limited institutional capacity for cultural legitimation. However, he is, above all, concerned with demonstrating how Catalonia's dependent status has made its culture vulnerable to symbolic violence and delegitimation, resulting in a crisis of representation by which Catalan discourses, practices, images and symbols have become invisible in mass culture, losing their capacity to represent society. It is the (in)visibility of Catalan theatre and performance culture that will be addressed in this chapter, as it is a theme that has generated a great deal of critical interest in recent years. For while on the one hand, as both Fernàndez and Crameri (2008) assert with confidence, Catalan theatre and performance cultures appear to have bucked the trend observed in other media, achieving a relatively high level of visibility locally, nationally and internationally, they have not remained impervious to the crisis discourse, but have been riven by often acrimonious debate over the structures and function of Catalan theatre. Indeed, it is telling that Sharon Feldman chose to entitle her ground-breaking study of contemporary theatre in Barcelona *In the Eye of the Storm* (2009) while nevertheless affirming that:

Catalunya is presently experiencing the most dynamic, extraordinary, opulent, and polemical period in its modern theater history. Barcelona [...] is the commanding hub of an energetic theater scene that over the course of the past two decades has witnessed an exuberant outpouring of new dramatists, a steady crescendo in theater attendance [...], and a continual increase in the international presence of Catalan directors, playwrights and companies.

(Feldman 2009: 10)

Feldman's profound analysis here and elsewhere (2002; 2004) of the dynamics of (in)visibility on the contemporary Catalan stage, by which local realities were elided in favour of more abstract spaces, explores how this particular geopathology mediates continuing questions of self-representation and identity, both interrogating and contributing to the construction of the kind of mirror in which contemporary Catalan culture might see itself. While she acknowledges how far 'the paradoxical presence of an "invisible Catalunya"' responds both to 'a desire [on the part of playwrights] to transcend their own cultural space' and to a more universalist or 'cosmopolitan yearning to project themselves and their work beyond local borders' (Feldman 2009: 43–44, 42), she does not go on to consider how far this is (in)visible for international audiences. Like Feldman, I am, of course, committed to investigating:

how does the Catalan stage negotiate the dialectic of the universal and the particular? In an age in which 'cultures overlap and mingle, enmeshed in a global struggle for self-determination',[2] how does contemporary Catalan theater participate in this struggle?[...] how can a play, playwright, performance, or director 'reveal' [...] or conserve markers of Catalan identity and, at the same time, transcend that identity to engender an international appeal?

(Feldman 2009: 26)

In the context of this volume, however, it is the latter question that is of most relevance, begging fuller consideration of what international audiences might actually see in Catalan performance culture(s). Thus, after this more general reflection on seeing Catalan theatre from the outside, I have chosen as a case study to look at contemporary Catalan directors' versions of *Hamlet*. For, while there have been various attempts to address the translatability of Catalan theatre and performance culture, these have tended to focus either on Catalan performance groups (Els Joglars, Comediants, La Cubana and La Fura dels Baus) or on the contemporary dramatic textual tradition (most notably, Josep Benet i Jornet, Sergi Belbel, Carles Batlle and Lluïsa Cunillé), often leading to a separation between the visual and the verbal that has contributed to confirm the sense that the Catalan focus on language as a differential marker of identity is somehow untranslatable for contemporary international stages.[3] Notwithstanding the growing number of volumes which have sought to represent the full gamut of contemporary Catalan theatre and performance culture (including George and London 1996; Delgado, George and Orozco 2007; Feldman 2009), there remain some troubling gaps (such as the scant critical attention paid to contemporary dance theatre), and only Maria Delgado has really begun to interrogate the interplay between verbal and visual traditions, in her work on Catalan directors (Delgado 1996, 2001, 2005) and in her reminder of the importance of the performative in *'Other' Spanish Theatres* (Delgado 2003).

Even so, it will no doubt appear perverse that a chapter on Catalan theatre in a book on theatrical culture in small nations should focus mainly on recent versions of one of the most translated texts of world theatre. Yet the choice is not as arbitrary as it might seem, for although for Lawrence Venuti 'a translated text should be a site at which a different culture emerges, where a reader gets a glimpse of a cultural order and resistency' (Venuti 1995: 305), it is also a zone of intercultural encounter in which meaning is negotiated between source and target languages, providing a two-way mirror in which to glimpse the cultural order and resistance of the source culture, too. When translated to the stage, this zone operates somewhat like the space of intercultural spectatorship envisioned by Bharucha, preparing 'one to see what cannot be understood through words. Through the smallest of details one can "listen" to how other parts of the body can "speak" [...] compensating for the inadequacies of one's comprehension' (2001: 196). Furthermore, Shakespeare's text, as can be traced in the whole genealogy of Shakespeare translation into Catalan from the nineteenth century onwards, is one that is precisely of interest to Catalan writers and theatre practitioners because of the relationship between the local and the universal perceived within his work, its symbolic power as an example of the imaginative capacity of a small, provincial, insular individual and nation to transform themselves into something of global cultural reach.[4] Above all, it affords a space in which to question and problematise the effects of the inequities of representation that accompany the small nation epithet, so that engagement in activities that might be perceived as normal in other cultures somehow become abnormal or even monstrous, requiring further justification or explanation.[5] By looking at four recent Catalan directors' *Hamlet*s I will address the key debate over the relationship between the particular and the universal in Catalan theatre and performance, negotiating the often contradictory readings of what constitutes the 'local' (and thus, variously, 'authentic', autochthonous, legitimate and/ or parochial, peripheral, exclusive) and the 'universal' (international, canonical, global and/or inauthentic, generic, un/anti-Catalan) as applied to contemporary Catalan Theatre. The main frame for my reading is that of visibility: both what makes a culture visible or invisible, and how far this is attributable to geopolitical factors such as size, language or cultural or political dependency; as well as the ways in which it represents its own desire for visibility. Perhaps unsurprisingly, the haunted mirror of *Hamlet* – a play known for its concern with ghosts and haunting – is one that places this dialectic on display; but, more particularly, as will be argued here, it is by learning to see the haunted mirrors of Catalan directors' *Hamlet*s that we can begin to perceive the different shape and changing structures of the Catalan theatre scene.

Catalan directors' theatre

If one were asked to list the names most associated with directors' theatre in Catalonia, so much so that for many they have come to stand for contemporary Catalan theatre on the international circuit, that list would almost certainly include Lluís Pasqual (1953–), whose work is included in dictionaries, surveys and studies of contemporary directors' theatre (see, especially, Delgado and Heritage 1996; Delgado and Svich 2002; Delgado 2003), Calixto Bieito (1963–), who became the veritable *enfant terrible* of European theatre (especially opera) in time for the new millennium, and increasingly Àlex Rigola (1969–), who as artistic director of the new Teatre Lliure in Barcelona endeavoured to forge links with the most important public theatres and festivals in Europe, and whose work is well-known in European theatre circles, if not so far within the United Kingdom. In some ways these directors, above all Bieito and Rigola, have come to share the mantle of the Catalan performance groups of the 1970s and 1980s, leading to the association of Catalan theatre internationally with a primarily visual if not always avantgarde and countercultural aesthetic. In others, they share the common characteristic of directors' theatre more generally, that is the tendency to focus on revivals, reimaginings and revisions of ancient or modern classics rather than on contemporary dramatic writing, leading in the Catalan cultural space to some criticism of their distortion and/or betrayal of Catalan theatre through their failure to represent local concerns and local authors.[6] All three directors have versions of Shakespeare in their repertoire: from the acclaimed version of *As You Like It* produced by Pasqual at the Lliure de Gràcia in 1983, to Bieito and Rigola's controversial and iconoclastic versions of *Macbeth* (2002), *King* Lear (2004), *Titus Andronicus* (2000) and *Richard III* (2005), among others.[7] All three have added versions of *Hamlet* to their curriculum vitae in the past decade, premiering in Catalonia within a four-year period (2003–2006). Here their versions will be discussed alongside that of one other director, Oriol Broggi (1971–), whose work in the past decade has often been cited as a counterpoint to that of the iconoclasts, and has come to stand for a treatment of the classics that is more reflexive and respectful, rooted in a relationship of faithfulness to the text, and the kind of close attention to language (here, in particular, the Catalan language) that is often felt to be the victim of the more visual imaginations of Bieito and Rigola. In other words, I will be using *Hamlet* as a mirror in which both to observe aspects of Catalan directors' practice, to detect and account for recent changes in paradigm, and to reflect currents in contemporary Catalan theatre, exposing aspects that are often invisible to the international gaze. This will ultimately bring us back to the problem of the relationship between local and global, and to an ethical haunting that is not just a question of the temporal relationship between past and present, but a spatial one regulating what can be seen, encountered and read on the global stage.

Hamlet in pieces ...

Let us start with the local and the anecdotal, based on what I have seen most recently of Catalan *Hamlets*. In May 2009 I was fortunate enough to see two different pieces of *Hamlet* on the same day: an open rehearsal of a few scenes from Broggi's *Hamlet*, with his company La Perla 29, on the ground floor of the Biblioteca de Catalunya (Catalonia's national library) in the centre of Barcelona, and an experimental Laboratory theatre piece entitled *El si el no Elsinore* at the relatively new former industrial warehouse space, the Nau Ivanow, in the peripheral district of the Sagrera.[8] In some respects, these were characteristic of the kinds of pieces of *Hamlet* traditionally available to a Catalan audience in the twentieth century: generally amateur or student versions of abridged sections of the play in translation or experimental actions based on specific themes isolated from the text.[9] Apart from such 'pieces' and the performances of foreign companies (dating back to the nineteenth century, with the Italian actor-manager Ernesto Rossi),[10] and more occasionally in Castilian, the only full performances of the play in Catalan were those of Terenci Moix's translation of the play in 1979–1980, directed by Pere Planella, with the actor Enric Majó, and Lluís Homar's self-direction in the role of Hamlet in 1999.[11] The difference was that since 1999, versions of *Hamlet* had been seen directed by three acclaimed Catalan directors alongside numerous international productions, from Lithuania, the United States, Germany, Russia, France, and the Ukraine, including directors such as Peter Brook (2002) and Thomas Ostermeier (2008) and companies such as the Wooster Group (2006).

I went back to see the Broggi *Hamlet* soon after it opened in June 2009 and was unsurprised, given the decision to hold some rehearsals open to the Catalan public, to find a self-consciously metatheatrical piece that reflected overtly both on the power of *Hamlet* and theatre in general and of this company and this theatre space in particular to communicate with its audiences. This power was framed in the programme and production paratexts as the capacity to tell the story of Hamlet plainly and simply, to communicate effectively with an audience using clear and accessible language, thus mirroring the translation poetics of the translator used for the production, Joan Sellent (2000).[12] Announced in English by the actor who played Horatius as 'The Tragical History of Hamlet Prince of Denmark', the group of seven players who gathered on stage at the beginning ghosted the Italian-speaking players who would appear later in the first part, and who played the *Mousetrap* in Italian, thus harking back to the nineteenth-century Italian companies who first brought *Hamlet* in performance to Barcelona. Hamlet's role within this interlude as an aspiring director ghosted the actor Jorge Manrique's own successful experiences as a director in the same season,[13] as well as the very rationale and approach to direction of Broggi himself as part of La Perla 29, alluded to through in-jokes and references included within the play, most obviously to the company's 2006 production of Tom Stoppard's *Rosencrantz and Guildenstern are Dead*.[14] Such ghosting added particular force both to Hamlet's criticism of the excessive histrionics of other companies (in Act I, Scene 3 and Act III, Scene 2) and to his description of the players in Catalan as 'el resum i la crònica del nostre temps' (the summary and chronicle of our time) as opposed to 'the abstract and brief chronicle of our time'. Indeed, given Broggi's own renown as a discreet and measured director, it is difficult not to associate the mirror up to nature speech with his own directorial philosophy, to the detriment of other directors, actors and companies, as was detected in audience complicity with Hamlet's criticism of those who are less respectful with the dramatic text.[15]

If it was clear that Broggi's intention was to offer his company's *Hamlet* up as a mirror to Catalan culture,[16] then it was a preeminently haunted mirror, to draw on the terminology used by Marvin Carlson in *The Haunted Stage*, in tracing the 'complex interweaving of space, memory, and cultural and geographical ghosting that is involved in the creation and ongoing use of "theatre spaces'" (Carlson 2003: 139). For Carlson 'any theatrical production weaves a ghostly tapestry for its audience, playing in various degrees and combinations with that audience's collective and individual memories of previous experience with this play, this director, these actors, this story, this theatrical space, even, on occasion, with this scenery, these costumes, these properties' (Carlson 2003: 165); yet, as he recognises in the case of *Hamlet*, drawing on a plethora of cultural and critical evidence and testimony, there are dangers in this haunting too: 'the density of its ghosting, culturally, theatrically, and academically [...] makes it a formidable, even daunting challenge' (Carlson 2003: 79). In many ways, the strategy used by Broggi, to foreground the many layers of ghosting through the range of overtly intertextual quotation employed in the play, may actually have contributed to provoke the main vein of criticism of the production, the lack of the kind of 'original' and distinctive vision of protagonist and play that one might associate with the many directors' *Hamlets* that inevitably haunted this one.[17] Furthermore, it was clear that there was not even full identification with the mirror he presented to Catalan culture, for aspects like the ghosting of the Italian players were misrecognised by some critics as an extraneous reference to the *Commedia dell'Arte*,[18] while the use of English by the ghost was read by Benach as an unflattering comment on the status of the Catalan language, which 'se supone es una caquita para los almas que flotan por las regiones celestes' (it seems is little more than a piece of shit for the souls that float through the celestial regions, [Benach 2009: 47]).

Haunted mirrors

Of course, this double bind can be seen as a feature of the doubleness of perception demanded by the theatrical experience in Carlson's account (50–51), or equally as a by-product of postmodernity, with 'the distinctive strain of Shakespearean representation of our time' tellingly identified by Dennis Kennedy as 'a tension between the decentring aesthetic and the desire to retain the plays as touchstones of traditional western culture'. 'Shakespeare,' he writes, 'has become more popular than ever before, the expression of his plays has become more complex, and old-fashioned historicism often exists next door to forms of postmodernism' (Kennedy 1996: 302). In the case of Catalan theatre and culture, as is liable to be the case in any minoritised, dependent or (post)colonial culture, the perceived need and demand for originality is in many ways stronger than ever, internally and externally, as a pre-requisite for visibility.[19] This is why some critics, like Josep-Anton Fernàndez, in *El malestar en la cultura catalana* (2008), but also Sharon Feldman (2002; 2004) and Carles Batlle (2004) in the case of theatre, have taken a politically and ethically committed stance on the relative invisibility of Catalan culture, showing how within a postmodern context, the lack of effective tools of legitimation produced by the rather ambivalent institutional frameworks imposed during the Spanish transition to democracy, has contributed to exacerbate the admittedly more generalised crisis in the production of shared myths and value in the case of the Catalan cultural field. As Fernàndez shows, this both makes it difficult to self-identify as Catalan because of the lack of effective mirrors, and can lead to alienation, denial and self-hatred through the presentation of distorted mirrors from outside. The director Lluís Pasqual, too, recognises a problem with identification and recognition in the Catalan cultural field, underpinning his call in 1997 for the creation of a new Teatre Lliure as part of a City of Theatre on Montjuïc, with his perception of the need for a place in which to see 'reflectida la nostra imatge d'una manera més rica, més complexa, més contradictòria, més noble, més innoble, més apassionant, més atractiva, en definitiva menys avorrida' (our image reflected in a way that is richer, more complex, more contradictory, more noble, more ignoble, more exciting, more attractive, above all, less boring [quoted in Feldman 2004: 161]). It is a problem Pasqual perceives more generally as contributing to the crisis in theatre at the end of the twentieth century, but one whose process of solution will be mirrored in the theatre it produces: '[I]f any human community, either consciously or unconsciously, begins to set the wheels of renewal in motion the theatre produced by that community will at the same time possess that new strength, and will be able to breathe life, not death, into the gestures which accompany its liturgy of celebration' (Pasqual 2002: 252).[20]

Before proceeding to scrutinise the 'haunted mirrors' presented by four Catalan directors' *Hamlets*, it is necessary to provide a brief genealogy of the particular use of haunted mirrors here. The concept was drawn initially from Josep Palau i Fabre's 1962 essay *El mirall embruixat*.[21] However, while this title is more commonly translated as 'the enchanted mirror', and no doubt owes much to both the hall of mirrors aesthetic that underlies Ramón del Valle-Inclán's formulation of a new theatrical genre in his coinage of the *esperpento*,[22] and to surrealist ideas as mediated by Artaud, my own partial mistranslation recognises both the importance Palau accords to *Hamlet* and draws his insights together with Carlson's much later – but exponentially mediated – formulations in *The Haunted Stage*. The epigraph to *El mirall embruixat* refers once again to holding the mirror up to nature, although this time as one in which 'cada generació i fins i tot cada època puguin retrobar llurs trets i llur caràcter' (each generation and even each age might rediscover its traits and its character). Furthermore, later in the text Palau draws on the *Mousetrap* as a model for the enchanted mirror offered by modern theatre, underlining the need for a mirror that looks at us too, that is capable of collapsing or inverting the relation between actor and audience.[23] Of the play within the play he writes that 'aquí, el teatre en el teatre, que sembla que hauria de ser l'element irreal, esdevé una mena d'alcaloide realista, perqué és grácies a ell que Hamlet pot constatar que la seva visió del fantasma i les paraules pronunciades per aquest no son una il·lusió; aquí la ficció li serveix per a controlar la realitat' (here, the theatre within the theatre, which seems like it ought to be the unreal element, becomes a kind of realist alkaloid, because it is thanks to it that Hamlet is able to confirm that his vision of the ghost and the words the ghost pronounces are not an illusion; here the fiction helps him to control reality [Palau i Fabre 1962: 85–86]). The scene's power, for Palau, is contained in the way in which it begins to multiply the mirrors offered to the audience, thus multiplying their own images, and leading to inevitable reflection on the limits of representation. Crucially, such a move away from the illusory theatre he associates with bourgeois realism depends on the 'llenguatge de la llibertat' (language of freedom), and can only be attained under particular sociopolitical conditions. In other words, here, as in an earlier essay, *La tragèdia o el llenguatge de la llibertat* (1961), his reading is coloured by the effects of the suppression of Catalan culture in 1940s and 1950s Spain and his own self-exile in Paris during the period.[24] This is important, for while in many ways Palau's haunted or enchanted mirror simply ghosts many other modernist approaches to world theatre, and in particular reflects the place of *Hamlet* in the theatrical canon – as theatre with a capital T – his association of the possibilities for such a theatre with conditions that did not pertain in Catalonia reminds us that Carlson's haunted stage can only function fully where there is space – a common ground – for the encounter between actor and audience. In terms of postmodern drama, that space has largely had to be created by directors' theatre, and it is the director, with or without the assistance of a dramaturg, who largely mediates the relationship between actors and audience. However, in the Catalan case, where access to a shared symbolic system was severely curtailed for nearly 40 years, there is a degree to which that relationship has had to be reconstructed and facilitated by other means, means that are visible in the celebrated performativity of Catalan culture (and in the international association of its theatre with performance groups), but the nature of whose haunting is more difficult to see, precisely because the limits between performer and audience has been blurred. The haunted mirror offered by *Hamlet* thus provides a frame in which to explore the relationship between Catalan directors and their particular locale, one in which Shakespeare's text took on a particularly emblematic character due to the specific history of Catalan theatre. At the same time it allows closer scrutiny of the kinds of mirrors Shakespeare presents to contemporary Catalan society, and how this has been understood and employed by different directors.

The directors then …

Calixto Bieito (2003)

First performed in August 2003, Bieito's production of *Hamlet* was developed with the Birmingham Repertory Theatre, taken to the Edinburgh Festival, and shown in Birmingham in September before being taken to Barcelona's Teatre Romea and then Dublin in October of the same year. While it was immediately recognisable as a Bieito production, it was his first time working with English actors on a Shakespeare play, leading to some reflection in the English programme notes on the characteristics of intercultural acting and performance, elsewhere explored by Delgado (2001; 2005) as one of the defining features of his work. In many ways, Bieito's *Hamlet* was the classic embodiment of the imagistic production, and also therefore mirrored the image of Catalan theatre that is most recognisable on international stages. He presented a very clear and accessible reading of the play based on the corruption of the court, which was ghosted through references to gangster films and contemporary music, fruit of an urge to get Shakespeare to mirror contemporary culture. Interestingly, what British critics found most disturbing was the mutilation of the text, rather than the overt gender violence that was rife throughout, with constant rapes and the reading of Ophelia's relationship with Polonius through violation of the incest taboo, introduced by Rachel Pickup (Ophelia) singing 'My heart belongs to daddy'.[25] In the United Kingdom, Bieito's *Hamlet* caused great controversy, although many recognised that it presented new insights and a fresh vision of the play. It was, in fact, far less controversially received by Catalan critics, although here the intercultural ethos of the play – recognised by Bieito in the particular demands (and pleasures) of working with British actors – might have contributed to mute some of the more vocal criticism heard when Bieito works in Catalan. The haunted mirror here is partly that of the monsters we often fear to see in our classic texts. But it also confirms the mirror of Catalan theatre that is generally seen internationally, with its focus on the visual and iconoclastic, thus confirming the limits of visibility of Catalan theatre.

Lluís Pasqual (2006)

Pasqual's *Hamlet* had been commissioned as one of the key productions for the Universal Forum of Cultures in 2004, in which case it would have joined a plethora of *Hamlet* pieces in the 2003–2004 season. When it was cancelled, there was considerable speculation in the press as to whether this was due to the usual budgetary problems, as the massive overspend on infrastructure led to a reduction in budget for content, or to the fact that Pasqual had elected to use a Castilian version for his production.[26] Whatever the reasons, his side-lining from the festival resulted in him leaving Barcelona to work at the Teatro Arriaga in Bilbao, where he planned to run workshops on the play, and prepared an ambitious project to play *Hamlet* and *The Tempest* alongside each other with the same cast, bringing a common focus on language, freedom of speech and violence (Larrauri 2006; Monedero 2006; Plana 2007: 42). The mirror he presented was thus a far more local one, embodied in his use of the charismatic actor Eduard Fernàndez as Hamlet, and one that focused far more on the excavation of the text, using his own, admittedly palimpsestic translation and relying on the power of his actors, with a minimal, empty stage to engage with the local Basque audience, in the context of a theatre that had been closed for many years. This would be seen as quite an audacious decision when he finally brought the play to the enormous space of the Sala Puigserver at the Teatre Lliure in Barcelona in the summer of 2006 as one of the star turns in that year's Grec Festival.[27] While Pasqual's return to Catalonia created great critical and audience expectation, reception of the plays was mixed, partly due to the use of Castilian rather than Catalan (and thus rather uneasy ghosting of the more resistant and defiant use of Catalan that characterised his years at the Lliure de Gràcia), but also because of the low key nature of the production, particularly when compared with the more spectacular opening sequence of *The Tempest* and the visual experimentation of The Wooster Group's *Hamlet* and Àlex Rigola's *European House*. The thematic link presented in the project was largely considered to have failed, suggesting that Pasqual was unable to mirror his vision of the plays. However, there were numerous ghostings of past productions and influences, in particular if read together and metatheatrically,[28] as we were encouraged to do by Francesc Orella and Anna Lizaran doubling as players in *The Mousetrap* and Prospero and Ariel in *The Tempest*. The message of theatre on a stage pared down to the bare boards (and an island whose contours were defined by pallets) is one that cut through the illusion to basic freedoms and the need for human dignity, to the core of the story and to the freedom of speech needed to tell it. Furthermore, the play ended with Hamlet's final words, 'lo demás es silencio' (the rest is silence), underlining its contained focus on the text and on language, while the decision to use a half-lit auditorium contributed to a heightened sense of actors and audience sharing a common space. Pasqual's basically humanistic vision about getting to the heart of the text and theatre has not really been seen on international stages, and this is arguably because it was not envisioned as a global spectacle. However, it also points to the limits of what we can be seen of Catalan theatre, as well as the relationship of Catalan culture with other peninsular languages and cultures.

Àlex Rigola, *European House* (2006)

In contrast, Rigola's 'Prologue to *Hamlet* without Words' was first showcased in the Festival Temporada Alta in Girona in the autumn of 2005,[29] but then was included in the programme for the following season at the Teatre Lliure on Montjuïc, where Rigola had been artistic director since 2003. From Pasqual's very text-based version there was, then, a shift within a few months to one that was almost entirely visual and that constructed its audience as rather knowing, cinematic *voyeurs*. The aesthetic was that of the comic book, with reminiscences of the imagistic, neon-lit German theatre directors with whom Rigola so identifies. Once again, it presented the mirror of Catalan directors' theatre that fits in best with the most prevalent visions of contemporary Catalan theatre, and a fresh vision of the text was offered – one which I have explored elsewhere (Buffery 2009) in terms of the complexity of its ghosting of past formulations of *Hamlet* in Catalonia – as claiming its originality from the mirror it presented to Western European culture. To some degree, both Rigola and the stage directors to whom he was indebted in realising this vision, Bibiana Puigdefàbregas and Sebastià Brosa, used their powerful imaging as a way of deconstructing the superficial iconoclasm of contemporary European culture; what they referred to as the 'falsa llibertat en què vivim la classe mitjana europea. Ho podem comprar tot, pero no som lliures d'esperit' (false liberty in which we the European middle classes are all living, in which we can buy everything but we are not free of spirit [Rigola 2006: n.p.]), where even 'Hamlet està atrapat per l'arquetip del jove revolucionari europeu. No se'ns permet ser originals en res' (Hamlet is trapped by the archetype of the young European revolutionary. We are unable to be original in anything [Rigola 2006: n.p.]). Yet the production also very clearly offered a haunted mirror in Palau i Fabre's sense, in the way in which its impact largely depended on the many ghostings of *Hamlet* buried in the minds of individual audience participants, which were subsequently shared in after-show discussion. Indeed, it was this that Víctor Molina saw as the greatest strength of the piece, celebrating the diversity of divergent opinions expressed by audience members: 'El teatro visual, que nunca es sólo visual, tiene como arte una relación con lo invisible que se deja ver, con una epifanía, que nos coloca en el centro de los orígenes griegos del teatro. Y eso nos causa preguntas. En hora buena' (Visual theatre, which is never purely visual, has at its centre a relation with the invisible that allows itself to be seen, like an epiphany, placing us at the core of the Greek origins of theatre. This makes us ask questions. And that's a good thing [Molina 2007: 50]). Its significance was not so much about communication, about translating the meaning of Shakespeare for contemporary European culture, as suggested in the programme notes, but about community, about making the invisible visible, producing a two-way mirror.

Oriol Broggi (2009)

And finally, we come to Broggi's *Hamlet*, the only one of these Catalan directors' *Hamlet*s that was actually in Catalan, in a language rarely heard on international stages, but always needing translation, always hidden behind the more recognisable visual idioms of the performance groups and iconoclastic directors. The translation used, that of Joan Sellent, had been commissioned for use by Lluís Homar, and thus ghosted a whole new approach to Shakespeare's language in Catalan, centred on performability and mediated by Núria Espert's recommendation to focus on getting the right version. In many ways, the play felt like it was trying to replay the whole of Catalan *Hamlet* history on stage, often playfully putting up mirrors to other aspects of Catalan theatre, but also drawing visual, musical, and multimedial cues from other *Hamlet* traditions and versions (including silent film, Brook and Meguisch, opera, lyrical and pictorial renderings of Shakespearian themes, different languages and cultures, and even the ghosting of Eduard Fernàndez's performance of the 'To be or not to be' speech while smoking a cigarette). La Perla's *Hamlet* celebrated its setting, using it to cradle its audience and make them feel part of the space; while the overt presentation of the company as actors, the presence of Broggi to welcome the audience into the performance space, the use of open rehearsals, as well as Manrique's Hamlet's direction of the players, presented a vision of the director less as a mediator than as a facilitator between actors and audience, who were all involved in sharing and creating meaning together. Nevertheless, the play also presented a Hamlet who increasingly turned his back on this role, as he was sucked into his own personal revenge tragedy – an individualist narrative that culminated in the pile of bodies on stage (thus ghosting the gore-fests unleashed by directors like Bieito and Rigola). Furthermore, the haunted mirror also contained the Catalan audience, representatives of whom were admitted and even asked to provide feedback during rehearsals, which contributed to reflect the dangers of individualism back on to them, pointing to the need for community and solidarity. This reminder to look outwards was brought home by the 'global' pictures of children at the end of the show, reminiscent of the photos in Plan International leaflets, who could have been from anywhere in the global South or could even have represented the cultural plurality of contemporary inhabitants of the district around this theatre space at the heart of the Raval.[30] When the actors came to life at the end, holding hands to troop out and then return for their bows, the image could just have easily evoked Unicef's hands across the world as more local Catalan dance traditions, such as the *sardana*, yet for me it also ghosted the more commercial images of the United Colours of Benetton.

Broggi's *Hamlet's* focus on a mode of direction that is more collective, democratic and facilitative both pointed to recent shifts in directors' theatre and reminds us of how far this remains invisible, at least in the case of smaller cultures, especially those in which the prospect that the rest is silence, with which Pasqual ends his reading of the play, is all too immediately experienced as part of the everyday. It reminds us of theatre's engagement in mediating and constructing new ways of seeing, but also perhaps the neocolonialism of excessive focus on the visual. It is a haunted mirror that demands that we see beyond the surface, to learn to hear and speak to other cultures; a mirror in which the visor effect (as theorised in Derrida's *Specters of Marx* (2003)) draws attention to our ethical duty to learn to speak *with* these ghosts. Rather than Carlson's celebration of a contemporary heteroglossic stage, which he sets in opposition to monolingual local theatres in *Speaking in Tongues* (2006), I prefer to imagine a vision of a heteroglossic *theatre*, where all languages might begin to be seen and heard on their own terms, rather than simply maintaining the oppositional frame of the dominant versus the subordinate, or the major versus the minor. Seeing Catalan theatre from the outside means exploring its changing relationship with other languages and cultures, assessing the problems that it presents for translation, and investigating the way in which it translates from other cultures. This is one thing I learned from studying the translation and reception of Shakespeare in Catalan; it was not just a work of translation studies, nor comparative literature, but a valuable opportunity to confront one version of universality, as a provincial Englishwoman, born in the same county as Shakespeare (a provincial Englishman, too, lest we forget, whose ability to compete on a global stage was ensured by sociopolitical conditions), with that of another geographical, linguistic and cultural context, and thus to learn to see my own culture from the outside. That is what I try to show my students when we try to see Catalan theatre in the classroom, though in reverse, as if in one of Palau i Fabre's haunted mirrors. Only then does the fragmentation of contemporary Catalan dramatic texts, the problems with communication and the motif of invisibility begin to become legible.[31] That is, we begin to understand the importance of language, and the need to make it visible.

Works cited

Barlow, P. (2006), 'Taboo or not Taboo: Voicing the Unspeakable. A Review of Hamlet by William Shakespeare, Directed by Calixto Bieito at the Birmingham Repertory Theatre, 18 September 2003', *Dramatherapy*, 28: 1, pp. 21–25.

Batlle i Jordà, C. (2004), 'De la realitat i el joc', *Pausa*, 20, pp. 69–76.

Benach, J.-A. (2009), 'El príncipe loco de Broggi', *La Vanguardia*, 13 June, p. 47.

Bharucha, R. (2001), *The Politics of Cultural Practice. Thinking Theatre in an Age of Globalization*, New Delhi: Oxford University Press.

Bruni, T. (2009), Interview with Oriol Broggi – 'Hem fet un "Hamlet" honest, no intel·lectual', *Avui*, 6 June, p. 40.

Buffery, H. (2007), *Shakespeare in Catalan: Translating Imperialism*, Cardiff: University of Wales Press.

——— (2009), 'Tròpics de Shakespeare: Orígens i orginalitat del Hamlet català', 1611: *Revista d'Història de la Traducció*, 1 April.

——— (2013), 'Negotiating the Translation Zone: Invisible Borders and Other Landscapes on the Contemporary "Heteroglossic" Stage', in Angela Kershaw and Gabriela Saldanha (eds.), Literary Landscapes and the Reception of Translation, special issue of *Translation Studies* (forthcoming).

Carlson, M. (2003), *The Haunted Stage: The Theatre as Memory Machine*, Ann Arbor: University of Michigan Press.

——— (2006), *Speaking in Tongues: Languages at Play in the Theatre*, Ann Arbor: University of Michigan Press.

Coca, J. (2005), 'Teatre polític', in Carles Batlle i Jordà (ed.), *I Simposi Internacional sobre Teatre Català Contemporani. De la Transició a l'Actualitat*, Barcelona: Institut del teatre, pp. 285–94.

Crameri, K. (2008), *Catalonia. National Identity and Cultural Policy, 1980–2003*, Cardiff: University of Wales Press.

——— (2009), 'Review of Shakespeare in Catalan', *Bulletin of Spanish Studies*, LXXXVI, pp. 133–134.

Delgado, M. (1996), 'Interview with Lluís Pasqual', in Maria Delgado and Paul Heritage (eds.), *In Contact with the Gods?: Directors Talk Theatre*, Manchester: Manchester University Press, pp. 202–219.

——— (2001), 'Journeys of Cultural Transfer: Calixto Bieto's Mulitilingual Shakespeares', *Modern Language Review*, 101: 1, pp. 106–150.

——— (2003), *'Other' Spanish Theatres: Erasure and Inscription on the Twentieth-Century Spanish Stage*, Manchester: Manchester University Press.

——— (2005), 'Calixto Bieito: A Catalan Director on the International Stage', *Theatre Forum*, 26: Winter–Spring, pp. 10–24.

Delgado, M., and Heritage, P. (eds.), (1996), *In Contact with the Gods?: Directors Talk Theatre*, Manchester: Manchester University Press.

Delgado, M., and Svich, C. (eds.), (2002), *Theatre in Crisis?: Performance Manifestos for a New Century*, Manchester: Manchester University Press.

Delgado, M., George, D., and Orozco, L. (eds.), (2007), 'Catalan Theatre 1975–2006: Politics, Identity and Performance', special issue of *Contemporary Theatre Review*, 17: 3 (August).

Derrida, J. (1994), *Specters of Marx, the State of the Debt, the Work of Mourning, and the New International* (trans. Peggy Kamzuf), New York: Routledge.

Feldman, S. (2002), 'Catalunya Invisible: Contemporary Theatre in Barcelona', in Brad Epps (ed.), special cluster in *Arizona Journal of Hispanic Studies*, 6, pp. 269–87.

—— (2004), 'Of Appearance and Disappearance: Theatre and Barcelona; Catalunya Invisible, Part II', in Brad Epps (ed.), Barcelona and Modernity, special issue of *Catalan Review*, 18: 1–2, pp. 161–80.

—— (2009), *In the Eye of the Storm: Contemporary Theater in Barcelona*, Lewisburg: Bucknell University Press.

Fernàndez, J.-A. (2008), *El malestar en la cultura catalana. La cultura de la normalització 1976-1999*, Barcelona: Editorial Empúries.

Foguet, F., and Santamaria, N. (eds.), (2006), *Una tradició dolenta, maleïda o ignorada. I Jornades de debat sobre el repertori teatral català*, Lleida: Punctum & GELLC.

—— (eds.), (2010), *La revolució teatral dels setanta. II Jornades de debat sobre el repertori teatral català*, Lleida: Punctum & GELCC.

George, D. (2007), 'Beyond the Local: Sergi Belbel and Forasters', *Contemporary Theatre Review*, 17: 3, pp. 398–410.

George, D., and London, J. (eds.), (1996), 'Introduction', *Contemporary Catalan Theatre: An Introduction*, Sheffield: The Anglo-Catalan Society, pp. 11–18.

Guibernau, M. (1996), *Nationalisms; The Nation-State and Nationalism in the Twentieth Century*, Cambridge: Polity.

Kennedy, D. (1996), *Looking at Shakespeare: A Visual History of Twentieth-century Performance*, Cambridge: Cambridge University Press.

Larrauri, E. (2006), 'Hamlet destruye destruyéndose a si mismo', *El País*, 2 February.

London, J. (1998), 'What is Catalan Drama? Language and Identity in Contemporary Catalan Theater', in Sharon Feldman (ed.), Homage to Catalan Theater, special issue of *Estreno*, 24: 2, pp. 6–13.

—— (2007), 'Contemporary Catalan Drama in English: Some Aspirations and Limitations', in *Contemporary Theatre Review*, 17: 3, pp. 453–462.

Molina, V. (2007), 'Del mundo interior al exterior', *DDT (Documents de Dansa i Teatre)*, 9: January, pp. 44–50.

Monedero, M. (2004), 'Lluís Pasqual no farà "Hamlet" al Lliure', *Avui*, 27 March, p. 49.

—— (2006), 'Pasqual i què fer amb la violència', *Avui*, 29 June, p. 41.

Orozco, L. (2007), *Teatro y política en Barcelona, 1982-2000*, Madrid: Asociación de Directores de Escena.

Palau i Fabre, J. (1961), *La tragèdia o el llenguatge de la llibertat*, Barcelona: Rafael Dalmau.

—— (1962), *El mirall embruixat*, Palma de Mallorca: Moll.

Pasqual, L. (2002), 'Afterword', in Delgado and Svitch (eds.), *Theatre in Crisis?* pp. 250–255.

Plana, D. (2007), 'Sóc Bessons', Interview with Lluís Pasqual, *DDT (Documents de Dansa i Teatre)*, 9: January, pp. 36–43.

Pujol, D. (2007), *Traduir Shakespeare. Les reflexions dels traductors catalans*, Lleida: Punctum & Trilcat.

Rigola, À. (2006), *European House*, Programme, Barcelona: Teatre Lliure.

Rossi, E. (1868), *Discorso improvvisato nell'Ateneo di Barcelona – La sera di lunedi 3 de mese di agosto del 1868, sopra il teatro di Shakespeare, e specialmente la tragedia Hamlet, sua interpretazione, sua esecuzionei*, Bilbao: Librería de Eduardo Delmas.

Sellent, J. (trans.) (2000), *Hamlet*, Barcelona: Quaderns Crema.

Udina, D. (2002), 'Ressenya de William Shakespeare, Hamlet, traducció de Joan Sellent', *Quaderns. Revista de Traducció*, 7, pp. 209–210.

Vall, T. (2004), 'Lluís Pasqual troba aixopluc per al seu projecte al Teatro Arriaga', *Avui*, 22 June, p. 44.

Venuti, L. (1995), *The Translator's Invisibility: A History of Translation*, London: Routledge.

Ytak (1993), *Lluís Pasqual: Camí de teatre*, Barcelona: Alter Pirene.

Notes

1   However you care to look at it, the body of Catalan culture can only grow if it can gain access to the market, if it can compete in the same field where the other normal bodies are taking part in the obstacle course. In a global context in which culture has become merchandise, and in a local context in which the Spanish culture industry colonises the Catalan market, the only possibility for the survival of Catalan culture is the adoption of strategies which allow it to compete on the same terms [my translation].

2   Feldman here quotes Guibernau (1996: 131).

3   Key texts in which this issue is discussed include George (2007), London (1998; 2007) and George and London (1996). Orozco (2007) gives a thorough-going account of the institutional prioritisation of Catalan-language theatre after the restoration of democracy, which led to the exclusion of more heterogeneous voices and practices. However, for a more balanced analysis of the sociopolitical context for late twentieth-century theatre policy in Catalonia, it is necessary to read her study alongside Fernàndez (2008) and Crameri (2008).

4   See Buffery (2007), especially chapters 2 and 3, for the symbolic value accrued by Shakespeare in nineteenth- and twentieth-century Catalan culture.

5   This was something encountered, for example, in responses to my own previous work on 'Shakespeare in Catalan' (Buffery 2007), considered by Crameri (2009) to require fuller explanation of the history and function of translation in Catalan culture. Such an explanation could have easily filled another volume; however, my point here is that it would not have been demanded had the target culture been French, German, Spanish or that of any other major European nation. Once more the Catalan cultural 'body' is unable to compete alongside other 'normal' bodies, to use Fernàndez's metaphor quoted at the beginning of the chapter.

6   For discussion of the insufficient acknowledgement of Catalan theatre tradition on Barcelona's stages since the Transition, see Coca (2005) and Foguet and Santamaria (2006; 2010) among others.

7   For a full list of Catalan Shakespeare productions to 2005, see Buffery (2007: 257–277).

8   In between, I got caught up in the celebrations of Barcelona Football Club's triple-cup-winning feat on the Via Laietana, arguably the most internationally visible phenomenon in contemporary Catalan culture, and one that has also brought reflection on models of management and direction, with Pep Guardiola representing the kind of collaborative teamwork that might be compared with Broggi's approach to theatre.

9   See Pujol (2007) and Buffery (2009) for fuller discussion of the history of *Hamlet* translation and reception in Catalonia.

10 The importance of Rossi for the nineteenth-century reception of Shakespeare in Catalonia can be gauged from the speech he was invited to give at the Ateneu Barcelonès, the most prestigious Catalan cultural centre of the period (see Rossi 1868).

11 Moix was one of the best-known counter-cultural novelists of the 1960s and 1970s, associated with Barcelona's Gauche Divine and the Catalan Gay Liberation movement. During the period in which he translated *Hamlet*, he became involved with Enric Majó and their relationship is reflected in the eulogies showered on the actor in the preface to Moix's prose translation (1980). Lluís Homar is one of the most celebrated contemporary Catalan actors, and has starred in recent films by Pedro Almodóvar, including *La mala educación* (2004) and *Los abrazos rotos* (2009).

12 Since being invited by Lluís Homar to translate *Hamlet* for his 1999 production, Sellent has gradually become the preferred translator of Shakespeare for the Catalan stage. He went on to translate *Coriolanus* for Georges Lavaudant's production at the Teatre Nacional de Catalunya (TNC) in 2002, with Homar as the main protagonist; *King Lear* for Calixto Bieito in 2004, and *Twelfth Night* for Josep Maria Mestres in 2010. His versions have been celebrated for their clarity and speakability, as in Dolor's Udina's review for the Catalan translation journal *Quaderns* (2002).

13 His version of Neil LaBute's *The Shape of Things / La forma de les coses* was premiered to unanimous critical acclaim at the Espai Lliure in Feburary 2009 and continued to tour in 2010, and he added a version of David Mamet's *American Buffalo* to his output in the 2009–2010 season at the Teatre Lliure.

14 Premiered at the Sala Beckett in May 2006, Broggi's *Rosencrantz i Gildenstern són morts* used actors of non-Catalan origin to play the main protagonists, leading to powerful reflection of contemporary experiences of exile, migration and diaspora.

15 This was a theme in reviews of the productions, such as Benach's celebration of an 'espléndido montaje' (splendid staging) in which 'no hay vulneración alguna del texto original' (no injury is done to the original text [Benach 2009: 47]).

16 Using Sellent's translation, this was expressed as 'un mirall on les virtuts s'hi puguin contemplar i els vicis hi quedin retratats, i on la imatge i el perfil de l'època s'hi reflecteixin fidelment' (a mirror in which the virtues might be contemplated and the vices be captured, and where the image and character of the age might be faithfully reflected), producing a subtle yet significant emphasis on the function of the mirror to reflect faithfully when compared with the original 'to show virtue her own feature, scorn her own image, and the very age and body of the time his form and pressure'.

17 While reviews of the production were generally positive, it was not considered to be as powerful as the version of *King Lear* he presented in the same space during the previous season (2008). Although Broggi himself acknowledged Peter Brook as a key influence on his work (Bruni 2009), and Manrique cited Chéreau and Branagh, it is arguable that the most important ghosting is that of Daniel Meguisch (1996) and his practice of intertextual quoting.

18 See, for instance, 'Tampoc sembla resolta l'escena de la representació que enfarfegada d'italià macarrònic queda forçada (per més homenatge que es vulgui fer a la *Commedia dell'Arte*)' (The scene of the play within the play does not work either, because the extravagant use of 'pidgin' Italian is rather forced [in spite of the intended nod to *Commedia dell'Arte*]). Furthermore, Benach dismisses the play's multilingualism as 'pijadas' (pretentious rubbish [2009: 47]).

19 As outlined earlier, Fernàndez (2008) offers a powerful and convincing reading of the Catalan cultural field in these terms, showing how the excessive obsession with quality, canonicity and, indeed, the literary in the cultural field is both caused by Catalan culture's weak position, meaning that it does not ultimately have power over the tools of legitimation, and responds to a misdiagnosis of its own postmodern and postcolonial condition.

20 It is interesting that Pasqual's own apparent rejection of Barcelona as a place for theatre, due to the 'enorme comercialització dels productes' (the enormous commercialisation of products [quoted in Vall 2004: 44]) as well as his now notorious disidentification with the model of Catalan identity propounded by former Generalitat president Jordi Pujol (Ytak 1993: 36–37) now appears to have been overcome with his appointment as the latest director of the Teatre Lliure in 2010.

21 The late Catalan poet, dramatist, essayist, cultural critic, translator and art historian is probably best known outside Catalonia for his work on Picasso, if not the more notorious anecdotes involving Antonin Artaud. While in exile in Paris in the late 1940s and 1950s, Palau penned a body of drama and dramatic theory that responded to the sociocultural and theatrical situation of his time, including a cycle of plays based on the myth of Don Juan and the books *La tragèdia o el llenguatge de la llibertat* and *El mirall embruixat*, published in 1961 and 1962, respectively.

22 Of course, the Galician writer's development of the *esperpento* itself bounces off *Hamlet* in its distorted mirroring of the gravediggers' scene from Act V, among other Hamletian themes reflected in *Luces de Bohemia* (*Bohemian Lights*).

23 The modern theatre with which he identifies is primarily the metatheatrical tradition associated with Pirandello, Lorca and the Theatre of the Absurd.

24 The military dictator Francisco Franco revoked Catalonia's 1932 statute of autonomy in 1938, going on to sanction the ferocious suppression of the Catalan language and culture in the decades following the Spanish Civil War. The Catalan language was banned from the public sphere, Catalan teachers and civil servants were redeployed in other parts of Spain, as part of a process of cultural 'purification', and anything that hinted at a differential Catalan identity was proscribed. Many Catalan writers, politicians and intellectuals went into exile to escape Francoist repression at the end of the war, and they were later joined by younger writers and activists who resented the lack of political and cultural liberties under the Franco regime.

25 The strange silence about the incest taboo has been read by Peter Barlow (2006) as a sign of denial and indicative of the 'ideology of containment' that has characterised British reception of Shakespeare's works.

26 Marta Monedero explains that he 'va abandonar per desavinences amb els responsables de les administracions involucrades al Lliure' (abandoned the production due to differences of opinion with representatives of the different administrations involved in the Lliure), going

on to clarify that the '[l]a cronologia d'infortunis continuà amb el fet que l'artista decidís que el muntatge fos en castellà, una tria que no va encaixar bé a la cúpula del teatre de Montjuïc' (the catalogue of misfortunes continued with the artist's decision to stage the work in Castilian, a choice that did not go down well with the powers that be in the theatre on Montjuïc [Monedero 2004: 49]).

27 Barcelona's main summer theatre, music and performing arts showcase, the Festival del Grec, was inaugurated, like the Teatre Lliure de Gràcia, in 1976. Both became symbols of the artistic freedom and community of the heady years of the Transition to democracy, and the period is remembered with nostalgia by many theatre practitioners.

28 Not only was it inevitable that Pasqual's presence in the new Lliure would evoke memories of his time at the Lliure de Gràcia, but its staging in the Sala Fabià Puigserver brought back the spectral presence of his long-time friend and collaborator and cofounder of the Lliure, who had designed the enormous, multi-purpose auditorium at the Palau d'Agricultura on Montjuïc. Indeed, both Pasqual and Anna Lizaran agree that 'Sí que m'emociono quan entro a fer teatre en una sala que es diu Fabià Puigserver' (Of course I am moved when I come in to make theatre in a hall named after Fabià Puigserver [quoted in Monedero 2006: 41]). The casting of Eduard Fernàndez in the central role ghosted Pasqual's previous work with the actor on *Roberto Zucco*, which was staged in the Palau d'Agricultura in the years before it was remodelled to become the new Teatre Lliure. Furthermore, many of the gestures used by the actor mimicked those of his director, leading his own mother to comment on their uncanny similarity (Plana 2007: 40). This multiplication of mirrors on a bare-board stage ghosted earlier productions by Pasqual, especially his celebrated work excavating the plays of Lorca in the 1980s and 1990s; and this ghostly presence was further detected in the casting of Marisa Paredes as Gertrude, an actress who in Almodóvar's *Todo sobre mi madre* (1999) appears with Pasqual rehearsing versions of Lorca. Above all, the plays together evoke Pasqual's most admired directors, Brook and Strehler, deliberately staging the two poles of his dramatic investigations.

29 This is a prestigious autumn theatre festival held in the northern Catalan city of Girona and the surrounding area, which often sees previews of productions that go on to be commissioned on Barcelona's stages.

30 The Biblioteca de Catalunya building is found in the old city district of the Raval, which was at the centre of José Luis Guerin's film *En construcción*. The library building was formerly a poor house, asylum and then a hospital, and its courtyard is now once more a makeshift shelter for homeless people.

31 I went on to develop this discussion of the grounds for embodied intercultural translation in an article entitled 'Negotiating the Translation Zone: Invisible Borders and Other Landscapes on the Contemporary "Heteroglossic" Stage' (Buffery 2013).

Chapter 5

Tales from the Wild East

Goran Stefanovski

When were we sexy?

I once discussed a topic for a speech with my friends from the Hamburg International Summer Festival. They suggested a provocative title: 'Why the East is not sexy any more'. I instinctively felt attacked. What? Me, *not* sexy? What could they possibly mean by that? Sexy how? Sexy by what criteria? 'Sexy' – What a cheap word! I looked at the question again. 'Not sexy *any more*?' This implied that we *had been* sexy before. Before when? When exactly were we sexy?

Could this mean that the East was sexy when it *was not* sexy? When it was struggling under the Stalinist yoke? And that it *is not* sexy now that it is trying to *become* sexy in the Western sense of the word? Was it sexy when it pretended that it was innocent and naive, and has stopped being sexy now that it pretends to be sophisticated and experienced? Was it sexy when it was passé and folkloristic and has it stopped being sexy now that it wants to emulate the West and catch up with the latest '-isms'?

My Festival friends are clever. Maybe their thesis was ironic, maybe deadly serious, maybe both. But they got me hooked. I started itching to say *something* on the matter. Something cynical, or something deadly serious or both. (My 'something' will zoom in on ex-Yugoslavia which is where I lived and what I knew best. I don't know how much my examples will apply to other Eastern European countries.)

Eastern Europe is desperately trying to reinvent itself and define its new identity. Its artists are waking up from a historical narcosis. They are rubbing their eyes, shaking off their delusions and resetting their memory. They are looking at the clock to check the time, feeling around to check the place. They are gazing at themselves in the mirror, bewildered. They wonder what to wear: 'What do I want to look like? Who am I?'

Most of the clothes on offer at the moment come from the fashion houses of the West. The Eastern European politicians are unashamedly parading in them. They feel proud to beg for money wherever they can smell it. They gladly change their countries' constitutions to meet demands from the European Union, the International Monetary Fund and the World Bank. They wholeheartedly embrace the global, multinational mode of operation and call it progress. Yet these same politicians no longer pay their artists. 'Sorry! No state control, no state money. We're all on the market'. Still, from these same artists, under the table, they tacitly expect a bit of nationalist purity, of searching for the roots, of the 'old-time religion'. They say: 'Yes, we have the new hardware now, but let's keep the old software. Yes, we *are* all on the market and we *have* sold our factories and our asses, but it's *your* job not to sell our hearts and souls.' So not only do the politicians keep their artists hungry, they also require them to sing.

No wonder some of the artists pine for the certainties of the 'ancien régime'. They say: 'At least the censors paid undivided attention to us and there was heating in winter. The dictates of the party weren't as ruthless as the dictates of popular taste. Socialist Realism wasn't any worse than Capitalist Realism.' This whole sweet-and-sour agony goes under the fanciful name of 'social transition', which is another name for spiritual rape.

And the West yawns. 'We've seen it all before. We went through that ourselves a hundred years ago. It's Oliver Twist primary accumulation of capital. Boring! You'll take a hundred years to reach our social democracy. By which time we might be off to the moon.' So the Eastern European artists seem to be doomed not only to undignified poverty at home, but also to being hopelessly out of fashion in the West, where they look for salvation. Insult added to injury.

My discussion with the Festival about the topic for the speech somehow came off the agenda with the beginning of the war in Kosovo. NATO bombed Serbia into oblivion, as if to jump-start it into modernity. Did that make us temporarily sexy again? I will never know.

How I lost my story

My name is Goran Stefanovski. This is the story of my life in a few short sentences. I was born in the Republic of Macedonia, which, at that time, was part of the Federative Republic of Yugoslavia. My father was a theatre director and my mother was an actress. I spent my first 40 years in Skopje as a playwright and a teacher of drama. I married Pat, who is English. We had two children and we were happy. We had a good story.

Then, in 1991, the Yugoslav civil wars started. Our lives took a sharp U-turn. Pat decided that the future of the Balkans was not going to be the future of our children. They moved to England. I started commuting between Skopje in Macedonia, where my secure past and my extended family were, and Canterbury in England, where my uncertain future and my nuclear family were. I started living between two stories. 'We've lost our story', I told Pat. 'No,' she said, 'the story has lost us'.

When I first arrived in England, as Sarajevo was burning, I met a well-meaning producer who wanted to cash in on my story and made no secret about it. She told me: 'Goran, you're an asset now. But it'll only last six months. You must hurry up.'

The six months passed. I didn't make my producer rich. Now I spend my days trying to work out the continuity between my two narratives and the artistic role of someone on the borderline. I patiently try to explain to my friends and relatives in Skopje that I haven't forsaken them forever and that I'm not living in the lap of luxury in the promised land of the West. I patiently try to explain to people in Britain that I am not a refugee bleeding-heart playwright with post-traumatic stress disorder. I have little success in convincing either side. They all seem to have strong ideas about who I must be. They have their clichés and stereotypes.

How my friends lost their story

So now I live in Canterbury, an olde worlde, touristy little town with a cathedral. On the main street there is a comics shop selling Americana novelties. In the shop window there is a life-size colour cut-out of a character from the popular television science fiction series *Babylon 5*. It is a picture of a creature with a big halo of flesh around her head. I know the actress behind this character. She is a friend of mine. Her name is Mira Furlan. She used to be one of the best actresses of ex-Yugoslav theatre, film and TV. She was the protagonist of our drama and the hero of our story. Now she is an alien. She has become one with the stereotype about Eastern Europeans.

Recently a friend came to see me in Canterbury. His name is Rade Šerbedžija. He was a legendary actor in ex-Yugoslavia. He was Hamlet. He was in countless films and new plays. He was the protagonist of our drama and the hero of our story. Rade is now an international star who gets parts in Hollywood films. As what? As a suspicious, Eastern European mafioso, an unreliable type, verging on the psychopathic. Hamlet has become a subsidiary character. The protagonist has turned into an antagonist. Rade has become an illustration of the cliché about Eastern Europeans.

We had a barbecue on a rainy English Sunday afternoon under an umbrella. We drank wine and talked about old times. Then I took him to see the photograph of his alien compatriot Mira Furlan. I looked at them next to each other – the two ex-heroes in virtual reality, outside their history and outside their geography and outside their story. I told Rade: 'We've lost our story.' 'Maybe we never had it', said he.

I can hear the yawns from the post-modernist gallery. 'Story. Continuity. Fate. Life. Death. Why are you Eastern Europeans so gloomy and pathetic and paranoid? Why can't you cheer up a little? Wake up! The world is a postmodern game!' Well, possibly, it is. Or, possibly, it can be – when it isn't a pre-modern mass grave.

What is a story?

A story is a narrative, an account, a sequence of events. It tells us who we are, who we have been, who we could become. It is an interpretation. Like identity, which is also a story of who we think we are, a constant negotiation and renegotiation of self. Like theatre, which likewise is a reflection, a vision of the world and oneself, a reading of the past and a projection of the future.

Let me make a few personal observations about how I see the differences between the Eastern and Western European basic stories, between the two master narratives. I hope that might throw some light on where my East is and how it came to be there.

Master narratives

Recently I saw a BBC documentary about Kosovo.[1] A teacher in a classroom in a Serbian school was telling his pupils that five hundred years ago a battle was lost against the Turks and that now it was their task to take revenge for it. This teacher was offering these children a narrative, a template for their identity. It was full of warriors, historical revenge, unsettled scores, sacred national ideals on the horizon. There was too much of my history in it.

My daughter Jana, who was six when we arrived in Great Britain, had stories in her first text book about a group of children who lost their dog on the London Underground. It was a funny story with a hint of magic in it. No history, no wars, no fixed identities. A global, open, decentralised, civic concept of the world. There was none of my history in it.

I kept asking myself which of these narratives was better for my daughter. And why should these narratives be mutually exclusive? And could there be a healthy balance between them? I needed urgent answers to these questions not only as a parent, but also as a citizen, not to mention as an artist.

Who is in charge of these narratives, anyway? They are written by civil servants in various ministries of education. (Apparently it took the German and French Ministries of Education ten years to finally standardise the school history books and decide how the subject was to be taught to children.)[2] These master narratives create the social context and intellectual discourse in which an artist operates. They are the centrifugal forces of society and culture. The artist can take it or leave it, but the context is there, like gravity.

Donald Duck v. Byzantium

I would like to examine these two different master narratives in their ugliest, most vulgar forms. Let me call the Eastern world Byzantium. It is a closed society, vertical, patriarchal, macho, rural, only one person at the top knows anything – it is a closely knit society, where you can never be lonely, but can never be left alone either. Social position is fixed; everyone has a nickname – your past, future and present are all a given thing. There is no democracy, no tolerance, no logical space for homosexuals – or women, for that matter. Individualisation comes at a deadly price. This is a world of ethnic fundamentalism. On one side, brothers are in eternal embrace; on the other, they are traitors and outsiders. This narrative is black and white and is only concerned with collectivist tribal issues. It allows primarily for a big National Theatre, casts of thousands, operatic reckonings. The Eastern European story is a tale of one lock and one key.

On the very opposite of this world stands Donald Duck. He lives in an urban, fast, global, consumerist, post-industrial society. He has no mother, no father, no wife, no children. He takes care of three nephews – God only knows whose they are. He sees his girlfriend from time to time, but then they go to their separate homes in their separate cars. Donald Duck doesn't belong to anything larger than himself. He is an individual par excellence. A loner in pursuit of happiness. He is like a cowboy in a saloon whose life depends on being quick on the draw. His narrative has no geography or history. It is splintered, fragmented, dispersed. Donald Duck is the bastion of political sterility and metaphysical failure.

Donald Duck enters Byzantium

What Eastern Europe has been witnessing in the last ten years is the entrance of Donald Duck into Byzantium. He walks with a swagger, and he brings with him his model of the world. (This model is primitive and unlike the Western European social democracy. It is a variety of cowboy capitalism with blazing guns. Or perhaps that is what it becomes when it reaches our shores.) Countless Western non-governmental organisations explain in endless workshops what should be done and how. The Eastern Europeans pay lip service and snigger behind their backs: 'Just leave the money and piss off. You ain't gonna tell me what to do.' Donald Duck comes with a stick and a carrot and the universal mechanism of greed and consumerism. 'Let's create chaos, and then establish our order. Let's create hunger and then sell our food. Let's make all the Chinese think they're worthless unless they drive one of our cars.'[3]

Eating salt

During our civil wars, CNN depicted us as tribes with complicated names and strange political habits. Against this backdrop were the groomed and coherent CNN reporters in pristine shirts, putting order into the chaos, explaining the mess in plain English.[4] Did it work? Western intellectuals would often catch me at international conferences and ask me in hushed voices: 'What exactly is going on down there?' So CNN did manage to make one thing clear: that we are incomprehensible. 'Don't bother to understand *them!*'

This is unfair and it hurts me. And I know how my mind works when I am hurt. I am ready, as the saying goes, to eat a kilo of salt. Let me shift gears here and stray from my chapter into a dramatic soliloquy in my atavistic voice: 'You think I'm incomprehensible? You ain't seen nothin' yet. I'll show you incomprehensible! Yes, I know I'm making a fool of myself and eating salt in front of you while you shake your heads. And I do it just to spite you. Just to damage myself. Because I've learnt in all of Dostoevsky that the only way I can prove I'm free is to work against my better interest. My Protestant wife will never understand this. She refuses to accept this as reasonable human behaviour. And I agree with her. But I only behave like this in unreasonable situations, under unreasonable pressure. Only when you step on my foot. So now you're telling me I'm an irrational monster. You, who've seen me before and who know I'm not usually this way. You, who've told me yourself how generous and hospitable and warm and bighearted and soulful I am. You say you're not happy with my story! You tell me I should change it? And unless I do, you will? You know what? Fuck you! How will you change my story? With a bombing campaign? With the Hague Tribunal?

With UN Resolutions? With bribes and blackmail? With theatre festivals? I don't think so. I'll change my story when I want to and if I want to. You think I'm not sexy? So what. As the poet said: "We're ugly but we have the music." Now you have me on the barricades! And this battle will go well into the next millennium. And in the one beyond it!'

Back to the chapter! Let me make one thing clear. I am ranting here against the ugly, invisible multitudes who make and maintain a cliché. I am attacking public opinions which are being discussed in bar and pubs. I am certainly not addressing here my friends in Frankfurt and Stockholm and Avignon and Kilburn who feel as much trapped by all this as I am. I'm not addressing the idealists who went to the Korčula philosophy school and who, in 1968, adored my ex-country,[5] and whose ideals now lie shattered just like mine. They can now see how the banks and international companies buy their own Western governments, as much as ours. Their world and my world are closer than ever.

Whose is the story?

Now that the wars are over, all we get on British television from time to time is news from the life of the British battalions over there. It is the story of 'our boys in the wilderness'. The story belongs to the storyteller. *Casablanca* is not about the Second World War in Europe and Africa. It is about a sexy American from New York. It is about an individual in pursuit of the American dream. It is about Hollywood and Disney. Excuse me, where is my place in all this? I don't mean private space, I mean personal space.

When Indiana Jones goes 'out there', he doesn't go to any particular history or geography. He goes to a jumbled-up Third World, full of greasy losers, mostly without a face, and mostly killed wholesale. Because Hollywood doesn't make room for geography and history, Eastern European artists don't feel properly represented. So they yearn to supply their history and geography. Their own map of the world. Their own compass. But here lies the trap which makes them obsolete. Their kids who go to the cinema are between 18 and 22 and they don't care about geography and history. They care about Indiana Jones.

How do you solve this impossible equation? In my part of town they say, 'How about I tie both your hands behind your back and we play basketball?'[6]

My map of the world

The West nurtured a granite conviction that 'no good could come from the East', that the story of the countries behind the Iron Curtain was one of a drab life, bleak aesthetics and secret police. This was a political projection created for the purposes of the Cold War. In Yugoslavia, we always cried for exemption, always wanted to prove we had 'our own way'. Perhaps we *were* an exception to the rule, but it was the exception which proved the rule. The cliché applied to us too.

(Of course I have these clichés myself. I have always been suspicious of anyone who plays rock and roll and is not white Anglo-Saxon or plays jazz and is not black. So I should not complain when I meet people who are suspicious of Eastern Europeans dabbling with the performing arts.)

So how was our story different from the cliché? What, if any, was our differentia specifica? Well, we grew up in the 1960s on our folk stories as much as we grew up on Kafka and Sgt. Pepper's Lonely Hearts Club Band. We enjoyed unrestricted travel abroad. We grew up on the Belgrade International Theatre Festival – BITEF. The Living Theatre came to Yugoslavia in 1968, when hardly anyone knew about them outside New York City. Grotowski, Brook, Bob Wilson were household names in Yugoslavia. We brushed shoulders with them. We believed that *we* sent them to the West. That they came to show us what they had first, and only then, after our approval, would they go and show it elsewhere. We were very pompous and arrogant. Almost sexy!

But, so what? Perhaps *because* the Yugoslav experience was this sophisticated it met such a shameful and violent end. Belgrade never really appropriated the novelties of its BITEF festival. It watched and observed, but it took little in. Under the veneer of Europeanism, it kept its Byzantine narrative intact.[7]

The deadly pull of the master narrative

The historical rhythms of Eastern Europe have been asynchronic with the West, particularly in the places which were under Ottoman rule. These societies never saw the Renaissance, Classicism or the Enlightenment, they never saw the Industrial Revolution, the Napoleonic Code or the social contract of Jean-Jacques Rousseau.

This arrythmia is a source of constant tedious comparisons and a permanent state of dismay. Our identity oscillates between deep inferiority and a lofty superiority. The inferiority is based on a sense of economic worthlessness. The superiority is based on a sense that we are the exclusive owners of Soul. (This is what even the two-bit Slav mafiosos believe. I personally can't see any differences between them and the two-bit mafiosos anywhere else.)

The luxury of artists in the West is that they can stay away from politics and still have ample space for discourse. In the East, because of the centralisation of society, there are no avenues for alternative discourse and no parallel spaces. Staying away from politics looks like retreating into autism. You can see productions, made smack in the middle of a historical earthquake, which bear no resemblance to that reality. They witness something else – a certain escapist solipsism of 'this is not happening, this is not here, this is not us'.

It does take a lot of courage to stay alive and make ends meet under the everyday pressure of that 'historical soap opera'. This courage cannot be appreciated from the outside. The Western observer pretends to know exactly what could be done in the situation, how these wrongs could be made right, and how this drama could be powerfully dramatised. (It's like watching football on TV and knowing how to score every time.) A Western novelist once said to me, 'I so wish I could live in your part of the world, then I would have a story.' That may be so, but she forgets that the chances are she would be so sucked into that story she would not have the time or the energy to even comprehend it, let alone articulate it in a novel form.

An unwanted story

So what was this lamentable lost story like in the performing arts of my ex-country? I believe it was authentic and genuine and pretty well articulated. In 1990 the Eurokaz Theatre Festival in Zagreb decided to show the Yugoslav 'performing arts story' as it then stood. Within the Festival there was a meeting of the Informal European Theatre Meeting or IETM. A whole new generation of young Yugoslav directors was presented to the Western independent producers. Their names were Dragan Živadinov, Vito Taufer, Haris Pašović, Branko Brezovec… These people were fearless in telling a story. I believe the story was sexy, as were the people who were telling it. As were the other, slightly older directors, like Slobodan Unkovski, Ljubiša Ristić, Dušan Jovanović… It was the story of our time and place and context, a pastiche, a tragi-comic tale of a world spinning between two mighty political grinding wheels. But the story failed to sell. The Western producers said it was hard to follow, difficult to file, they said it did not match Western horizons of expectation.

So the story went to the dogs together with the storytellers. Some of them became ideologists of political regimes, some ministers of culture. They were all sucked in by the centrifugal forces of their respective master narratives. Perhaps the Western producers (and here I mean not only theatrical, but also political) could have tried to create a context, to adjust the horizon of expectation to the story, and not vice versa. Perhaps, just perhaps, if that story had been recognised and supported, there would not have been the war which demolished it.

And now, after the rivers of blood, the question arises again: 'Wo ist Osten?' Well, there was a time when the East (at least my corner of the East) was screaming, 'Here we are!' and the West replied, 'We can't see you. You're not where we expect you to be. Be somewhere else, so we can see you.'

But that is all history now. And there's no use crying over spilt milk. I know there was nothing personal in it, amigos! It was strictly business!

What to do?

It is street wisdom in the Balkans that it is impossible to be born and to die in the same country. Within one's lifetime, the house will fall on your head and you'll have to start building again. 'The constant repetition of the same.' It is a given, like a natural disaster.

The Eastern European theatre is stewing in the pressure cooker of political turmoil and is undergoing a tectonic shift of identity. It is consoling itself that real artistic birth is only possible in the crucible of historical pain. (And, to be fair, there is the towering Western success of the films of Kusturica and Manchevski and the music of Bregović which the Eastern European performing artists can strive to emulate.)[8]

The Eastern European performing artists will have to snap out of their amnesia and remember that it was their own convoluted society which, in a spasm at the turn of the century, spurted out Chekhov, Malevich, Stravinsky, Eisenstein, Nijinsky, Harms, Vvedensky and Bulgakov. The same names which the ever-so-flexible West appropriated as its own. And so it happened that the East which came up with these names became known as the Wild East. And the Wild West, which came up with Wyatt Earp and Calamity Jane, became the suave and cool proprietor and guardian of modernism.

The Eastern performing artists have some old-fashioned and lonely homework ahead of them – to find their voices, remember their names, regain their self-assurance, reclaim their space and recognise their continuity. They have to earn their stories and make them their own. For whatever these stories are worth. And however sexy they may, or may not, be.

Afterword: Collaborate?

In the early years of my living in two worlds, I was lucky enough to work on a number of European projects. I worked with a friend, a partner, a producer, an Italian American living in Sweden, called Chris Torch. Our projects included collaboration with various Eastern European artists, but were primarily co-financed by Western European countries and aimed at Western European audiences.

This packaging caused confusion and consternation in some quarters. I witnessed a series of misunderstandings and dramatic ironies, traps and pitfalls, hits and misses. Chris Torch believed he was championing the cause of sharing cultures, crossing borders, re-mapping, making sense of the new European challenges. He believed he was a mobile cultural operator, a pioneer of European integration, citizenship and community-building.

But on the ground, I heard libels, loud and hushed, aimed against him, but which reflected against me as well. Some folks saw him as a cigar-smoking slave driver. I heard the terms 'cultural imperialist', 'multinational trickster', 'globalisation shark'. Both sides of the fence suspected him as someone who buys cheap artistic labour in the East and sells it for profit to the West. Many people didn't care what the performances or the actual artistic articulation were like. They hated the idea on principle.[9]

I was bewildered. Suspecting my friend, Chris, of all people? The actor from the Living Theatre, the ultimate anarchic wild bunch of the 1960s?[10] The man who founded a theatre commune in Stockholm? I thought he was cool. But other writers didn't, they told me to be careful. Especially as he was working with me and not them.

One day there was a meeting between some Macedonian actors and Chris in Skopje. They asked how much money they would be paid for their work. He answered it would be standard European wages. One of the actors sniped, between his teeth, 'I can find that kind of money in the street.' He was lying. There was no money to be found in the streets of Macedonia. Chris said, 'I thought you wanted to make theatre and not look for money in the streets.'

This conversation has stuck with me over the years. To this day I wonder about the mindset of my actor friend, his manoeuvre, his mental calculation. He probably thought something like this: 'I know I am worth little in market terms and I am quite resigned to that fact. But now here is this guy who comes *from* the market place and is showing interest in me. Why? What's in it for him? Maybe I'm worth something after all. What if I'm priceless and don't know it? This is a conspiracy. I won't sell. I'll wait for better offers.'

One day in 1995 Chris and I went from one Macedonian theatre to another trying to garner interest for our multi-ethnic project. We were working on a remake of Euripides' *Bacchae* where the Bacchantes were all male. We wanted actors of Macedonian, Turkish and Albanian ethnic origin to dramatise the reality on the ground. We went from door to door, from the Macedonian National Theatre to the Drama Theatre to the Theatre of Turkish and Albanian Nationalities, inviting them to collaborate.

This turned out to be an explosive proposition. 'Collaborate! We've never collaborated before. We're suspicious of each other, we protect our interests, we're almost enemies. What do you mean, collaborate? We are trying hard to rid ourselves of those socialist-realist ideas and you want to sell them back to us? Are you trying to sell rope to the family of a hanged man?' Incidentally, that was the very day when there was the assassination attempt on the life of the President of Macedonia, Kiro Gligorov.[11]

It became obvious to me that one humble producer like Chris Torch can shake the very centre of a small, national, macho, patriarchal cultural mindset. That one person can become a screen for every passion and fear, desire and paranoia which happens to be flying around. Like a lightning rod, that one person attracts whatever energies and anxieties people have about the world and themselves. With the best intentions of soft-core integration you can go straight to hard-core nationalist hell.

This mindset is a maze of contradictions, half real and half virtual, half genuine and half artificial. It is so convoluted that it is difficult for outsiders to understand it or probe into it. It is a mindset of bi-polar divisions, a melodramatic world of black and white. You're either my bosom friend and I love you to death or else you are my arch enemy and I'm at war with you. The changes from one pole to another are swift and volatile and you never see them coming. It is slippery ground. Mercurial stuff.

Hotel Europa

I conclude with an account of a project where I personally tried to answer the question of 'What to do?' It was a narrative which came out of the crack between the old narratives which had not yet left and the new narratives which had not yet arrived.

In the year 2000 I wrote the script and worked as a dramaturg on a project called *Hotel Europa*. It was a complex enterprise which took over a year to prepare and perform. I originally wrote the concept and the first draft of the script, which was followed by a meeting with all directors, where the material was discussed. Afterwards I wrote the further drafts of the script.

The project was produced by the above-mentioned Chris Torch of Intercult, in Stockholm. He is an American and a naturalised Swede, a real artistic and human live-wire force.

The production was directed by nine directors and performed by 25 actors from several mainly Balkan and Baltic countries. Every director worked with their own team and their own style. Some scenes were written as drama, some as dance librettos and some as installations. Some scenes mutated from their original version to suit the style of the director and the actors.

'Europeretta' was directed by director Viesturs Kairišs and visual artist and designer Ieva Jurjane, from Latvia. 'Do Not Disturb' was directed, mainly as a dance piece, by choreographer Matjaž Farič from Slovenia. 'One Night Stand' was directed by Oskaras Koršunovas from Lithuania. 'Room Service' was directed by Dritëro Kasapi from Macedonia. 'Hotel Angels' was directed by Piotr Cieplak from Poland. 'Maiden Voyage' was directed by Ivan Popovski from Russia. 'The Empty Rooms' were installations staged by the Art Action Group 'Škart' from Yugoslavia. 'The Grand Hotel Casino Europa' was the central scene directed by Nedyalko Delchev from Bulgaria. The Roving Characters were directed and performed by local artists from the co-producing parties and countries.

The production was performed in five European cities in the summer of the year 2000. It was performed in specially adapted huge spaces of 'derelict buildings'. In Vienna it was co-produced by Wiener Festwochen and performed at the Kabelwerk, an old cable factory. In Bonn-Bad Godesberg it was co-produced by the Bonner Biennale and performed in an empty former department store in the centre of town, Das ehemalige Hertie-Kaufhaus. In Avignon it was co-produced by Festival D'Avignon and performed in the Usine Volponi, a warehouse 20 minutes bus ride from the old walled town. In Stockholm it was produced by Intercult and performed at Medborgarhuset, a huge public building in the centre of the south part of town, which includes a swimming pool. In Bologna it was co-produced by the City of Culture of Bologna and performed in a building which used to be an aquarium.

Sören Brunes did the overall complex production design. The project resembled a military operation and required military precision. An audience of 300 would enter the building for an opening scene. Then it would be split into six groups of 50 and taken to separate rooms for individual scenes. There were six scenes going on in synchronicity, each lasting roughly 15 minutes. After each scene a Roving Character would lead the audience from one room to another, where another scene would start. Groups of audience members would sometimes brush shoulders with each other in corridors during these journeys.

It was extremely important for these transitions to go smoothly, which was not easy at the best of times. In the middle of the performance all of the audience would gather in a big 'banqueting' hall for the longer central scene. After this, there would be further journeys of the audience for the remaining scenes. This means that people saw the production in a different order of scenes and consequently with a different narrative flow.

All these years later I am still reeling with excitement when I think of the sheer sweeping breadth of the *Hotel Europa* project.

In 2009 the script was published in New York in *New Europe, New Voices,* an anthology of plays edited by Malgorzata Semil and Bonnie Marranca, by the Performing Arts Journal, New York.

Works cited

Goulding, D. J. (2002), *Liberated Cinema. The Yugoslav Experience 1945–2001*, Bloomington: Indiana University Press.

Iordanova, D. (2001), *Cinema of Flames. Balkan Film, Culture and the Media*, London: BFI Publishing.

Klaic, D. (1997), *Reform or Transition: The Future of Repertory Theatre in Central & Eastern Europe*, New York: OSI.

——— (2008), 'National Theaters Undermined by the Withering of the Nation State', in Stephen Wilmer (ed.), *National Theaters in Europe*, London: Palgrave, pp. 217–227.

——— (2009), 'Post-Yugoslav Theater Exile: Transitory, Partial and Digital', in John Neubauer and Marcel Conis Pope (eds.), *Exile and Homecoming: East-Central European Writers in a Twentieth-Century Diaspora*, Berlin: De Groyter.

Marciniak, K. (2003), 'Transnational Anatomies of Exile and Abjection in Milcho Manchevski's Before the Rain', *Cinema Journal*, 43: 1 (autumn), pp. 63–84.

Norris, D. (1999), *In the Wake of the Balkan Myth*, London: Macmillan Press.

Ramet, S. P., and Adamovic, L. (eds.), *Beyond Yugoslavia: Politics, Economics and Culture in a Shattered Community*, Boulder, CO: Westview.

Ravetto-Biagioli, K. (2003), 'Laughing into an Abyss: Cinema and Balkanization', *Screen*, 44: 4 (winter), pp. 445–464.

Notes

1   The BBC documentary *Moral Combat: Nato at War* was transmitted on Sunday 12 March 2000 on BBC2.
2   See Claude Carroué's article, 'History Textbooks Build Bridges to Understanding', in *Worlds of Education,* Issue 27, September 2008.
3   *In the Wake of the Balkan Myth* (1999) by David Norris offers a large historical and cultural overview of the Balkans.
4   CNN, 1st October 1998, http://edition.cnn.com/WORLD/europe/9810/01/kosovo.02/.
5   The widely popular Korčula Summer School on the island of Korčula in the Adriatic, was organised by the Praxis group, a Marxist humanist philosophical movement. It originated in

Zagreb and Belgrade in SFR Yugoslavia in the 1960s. From 1964 to 1974 they published the journal *Praxis*, renowned as one of the leading international journals in Marxist theory.

6 Dina Iordanova's *Cinema of Flames* (2001) presents an in-depth study of how Balkan film 'story tellers' have been dealing with these equations.

7 For a brilliant and comprehensive analysis of post-Yugoslav theatre, see essays by Dragan Klaic listed in the bibliography.

8 See analysis of Manchevski's film *Before the Rain* in Katarzyna Marciniak's 'Transnational Anatomies of Exile and Abjection in Milcho Manchevski's *Before the Rain*' (2003).

9 For an excellent analysis of this process of 'Balkanization', see 'Laughing into an Abyss: Cinema and Balkanization', by Kriss Ravetto-Biagioli (2003).

10 During the 1950s and early 1960s in New York, The Living Theatre pioneered the unconventional staging of poetic drama. In the mid-1960s, the company began a new life as a nomadic touring ensemble. In Europe, they evolved into a collective, living and working together towards the creation of a new form of nonfictional acting based on the actor's political and physical commitment to using the theatre as a medium for furthering social change. The landmark achievements of this period include *Mysteries and Smaller Pieces, Antigone, Frankenstein* and *Paradise Now.*

11 On 3 October 1995, the President of the Republic of Macedonia, Kiro Gligorov, was the target of a car bomb assassination attempt in the capital Skopje. He was seriously injured. The perpetrators are still not known, 15 years later. Gligorov was succeeded as president by Boris Trajkovski, who tragically died in a plane crash in 2004.

Chapter 6

A National Theatre in New Zealand? Why/Not?

Sharon Mazer

Culture is a sort of theatre where various political and ideological causes engage one another.

(Said 1994: xiv)

N ew Zealand does not have a national theatre as such, or even a singular, official theatre history. Instead, there have been a number of theatrical movements, arising over time and interwoven in layers, like the tukutuku panels that adorn the walls of Māori meeting halls. Rooted in the colonial past, almost entirely imported and explained from the British perspective, and now deeply influenced by film, telemedia and the Internet, theatre has only recently come to be seen as essential to who we are and how we communicate with each other, and the world, as New Zealanders. It seems past time to institute a national theatre – or perhaps two, one representing Māori and one representing the rest of us. But why? And why not? This chapter explores the question of national theatre(s) in the postcolonial context, looking at how, and to what possible effects, the loosely interlocked threads of New Zealand's theatres might be tied into a wider cultural frame.

Of course, the question of a national theatre in New Zealand (as elsewhere) both presupposes and proposes a cohesive national identity – or at least an image of this country that is recognisable to a substantial portion of the population and can be offered up as a nation-representation abroad. It might even seem easier to achieve this goal in a small country, isolated at the edge of the South Pacific, than in more trafficked and (presumably) diverse parts of the world, and it seems a necessary step in the process of moving past the colonial period towards independent nationhood to establish a national theatre. It is a commonplace of theatre history, after all, to represent the emergence of a theatrical 'golden age' as the way the relationship between language and culture is consolidated into a more or less unified idea of national identity. (Indeed, this is the way I teach theatre history here: Greece, Rome, England, Italy, Spain, France, Germany, Norway, Sweden, the United States, New Zealand …) But a small nation is, in many ways, like a small town, at least as is likely to provoke its citizens to claim essential differences as to incline them towards hegemony.

The beginnings of a theatre distinctive to New Zealand are tied to the pioneering plays and performances of Bruce Mason (1921–1982) and Mervyn Thompson (1935–1992), who between them engineered the shift to New Zealand stories and voices. Their signature performances – Mason's *End of the Golden Weather* and Thompson's *Coaltown Blues* – are significant in their original settings for the way they translated their coming-of-age narratives into paradigmatic tales of New Zealand's coming of age as a nation still bound to Britain, but separated by geography and time, run aground – or, as George Parker says 'beached' – in the history of discovery, settlement and social awakening. These solo performances about coming to know themselves as New Zealanders conflated the personal and the social in a way that might be seen as a template for the past twenty years of performances about the tension between cultural identities – especially those wrought from living outside the English/Māori (i.e., coloniser/colonised) binary – and national identity.[1] In Edward Said's words, 'nations themselves *are* narrations' (1994: xiii).

It is impossible to think of a national theatre in New Zealand without thinking of *the* National Theatre (London) as a source both of aspiration and of limitation. The idea of national theatre, like the idea of nation, is not only an ideal; insofar as a national theatre may be seen to enact an idea of nation, it's an ideological construct, one that might be seen to be especially problematic in a postcolonial context.[2] Still formally tied to Britain and yet bound by the Treaty of Waitangi, Aotearoa New Zealand – as the name suggests – is not so much a bicultural country as a hybrid nation, as such no longer colonial, really, and yet not quite postcolonial, officially bicultural but both less and more than that in practice. In the twenty-first century, Aotearoa New Zealand as a nation-ist idea exists if not dialectically, then dialogically between Māori and Pākehā, between its indigenous peoples (tangata whenua, the people of the land) and the descendents of its early British settlers.

But these islands are full of other others: Pacific Islanders, East and South Asians, Africans, Europeans, and even Americans (such as myself). Many of us have washed up here with our own, at times fierce, conceits about the relationship between what might be seen to be our originary homeland(s) and this land, creating floating communities, islands of identity in what is supposed to be the post-identity politics era. The past twenty years here have seen the emergence of a series of signature theatre works, each signalling a new string of hyphenated identifications – Samoan-New Zealander, Chinese-New Zealander, Indian-New Zealander, Jewish-New Zealander, and so on – demanding inclusion while resisting any notion of a seamless integration into the existing Māori / non-Māori binary. As David O'Donnell has observed, writing as someone whose theatre work is woven into the narrative of New Zealand's theatre history: 'There has been a move away from theatre as an expression of a collective identity to theatre which not only expresses multiple identities, but questions any notion of a fixed identity' (2007b: 25).

In this small nation we seem sometimes to be perpetually remaking ourselves into ever smaller mini-nations-within-the-nation. Perhaps this is an inevitable development in postcolonial New Zealand. After all, the idea of theatre is, itself, historically a European construct, an instrument of colonisation in its own right, as noted by Edward Said, among many others: 'The great cultural archive [...] is where the intellectual and aesthetic investments in overseas dominion are made' (1994: xxiii). As such, it inevitably establishes a frame that has been extended (to my mind unconvincingly) to the diverse performance practices of non-European nations over the past century, and in the postcolonial context, further complicates any consideration of a national theatre in Aotearoa New Zealand.

It must be admitted, before I proceed further, that my way of thinking about the question of a national theatre in this small nation has been predicated by my own arrival here, over 15 years ago, from New York City. One of the last productions I saw on Broadway was the Almeida Theatre Company's *Medea*, directed by Jonathan Kent and starring Diana Rigg. The first production I saw in Christchurch was the Court Theatre's *Medea*, directed by Elric Hooper and starring Geraldine Brophy. The production I saw in New York was emphatically asymmetrical, striking for its sense of physical scale – the rough rusty fortress walls towering over the actors, the apparently vast sands stretching the full width and depth of the stage – and the atonal scale plumbed by the chorus – three darkly draped women, moving in oblique patterns as if already in mourning for the soon-to-be-murdered king, princess and children.

What I saw in Christchurch was revelatory in its own way. It was as if the production I'd seen in New York had been uplifted from the vertically vast Broadway theatre, its imposing structure diminished, re-engineered into something resembling large heating ducts and pressed into horizontality in order to squeeze into the wide but short and shallow Court Theatre stage; the shadowy, ominous women of the chorus were converted into something babushka-esque, their song made harmonic, pleasing to the ear. For me, in my fresh-off-the-plane arrogance, this became a paradigm for New Zealand theatre: not simply derivation, more simulation than imitation, driven not so much by a desire for artistic epiphany as for conformation, a settling into bourgeois complacency. Why go elsewhere? Here we are as good as there. Or at least, what we take from there can be bent to fit the room in which we find ourselves, and if such strainings and stoopings often lead to Alice-in-Wonderland-like contortions, then what we see as a result is still more evolutionary than revolutionary.

The Court Theatre was founded in 1971, by Mervyn Thompson and Yvette Bromley, at a critical point in New Zealand's coming to see itself as a country, still attached to but increasingly distinct from its origins as a British colony. It wasn't the only theatre founded in the hopes of establishing a theatre that could represent the lived realities and cultural aspirations of New Zealand,[3] but it is the one that survived more or less intact, and it now claims primacy as the sole professional producer to maintain a core company year-round. From the start, the theatre teetered between two poles. As its name suggests, the Court Theatre Christchurch was deliberately modelled on the Royal Court Theatre in London – 'Britain's first national theatre company' with the word 'Court' reflecting, at least superficially, Christchurch's enduring affection for its not-so-distant colonial past (Royal Court Theatre 2010). In the beginning, the Court Theatre's founders drew inspiration from the Royal Court's relative radicalism: its commitment to presenting performances of plays that were driven by contemporary, local social issues, plays that challenged not only the status quo outside the theatre but also the hegemony of the 'great play' – the grandness of the classical repertoire – in British theatre of the time.

By all accounts, early productions by Mervyn Thompson, in particular, followed this radical impetus, but as the Court Theatre settled into the Arts Centre, it also settled into a less controversial mode of playmaking. It presents seasons that balance 'great plays' (i.e., the classics), current international successes and an annual summer musical, with one or two New Zealand plays – usually comedies, most often by New Zealand's most successful playwright, Roger Hall, who has been charting the foibles of the middle class here for many decades. That is, the Court's repertoire works much like the regional theatres of the US, or the National Theatre in London, albeit without the degree of critical self-reflection these theatres often claim to provoke. The Court does a wonderful job of pleasing its audience, making them feel at home in the theatre, reassuring them that as far from the bright lights of London or New York as they are here, they are seeing 'the arts of theatre [performed] to the highest international standard' (Court Theatre 2010). When it produces New Zealand plays – for example, a Roger Hall play, such as *Dirty Weekends* (a paean to the addictive pleasures of gardening, from one generation of middle-class New Zealanders to the next) – Christchurch audiences fill the theatre with the laughter of recognition, and they come prepared to be jolly, even when there's not so much to laugh about, as I observed during a recent performance of Gary Henderson's *Home Land* (an elegy for the 'Southern Man,' set in Otago).

The Court, it seems, is not so much a national theatre as a neighbourhood playhouse, one that stages a sense of being at home in the world without risking the safety of our seats. There's even a place for those other others, in the Court's smaller studio theatre, which these days is called The Forge and has been recently dedicated primarily to producing plays by New Zealand playwrights, including a number of Pasifika artists. As with regional theatres in the US, and the National and Royal Court theatres in London, the geography of the Court Theatre in Christchurch thus reproduces dominant cultural values on the mainstage while preserving room at the margins for the more marginal. The tangled threads of New Zealand's diverse cultural narratives are smoothed into a soothing theatrical framework that preserves, at its heart, the aspirations of its leading citizens – like a piano carefully transported by ship to be given pride of place in the settler's parlour. The odd notes that are sounded as a result are not necessarily heard as such by those whose ears are tuned as much by nostalgia as by lived experience.[4]

Theatre in a small, postcolonial nation such as New Zealand can, it seems, be seen to enact a kind of 'rite of return' in which the newcomer (or newer comer) stages a process of coming to terms with the here and now within the set frame of the there and then. This is true not only of explicitly Britophilic theatres such as the Court, but also of many of the smaller theatre companies that dot New Zealand's artistic landscape. How can it not be, when the very framework of the theatre always already hearkens back through the arc of European theatre history which defines it and gives it value? My Canterbury colleague, Peter Falkenberg, rehearsed this issue in a recent issue of *Theatre Topics* from the perspective of a European theatre director who, as founder and artistic director of the Free Theatre, has been making avant-garde theatre in Christchurch for the past 30 years (Falkenberg 2005: 39):

Coming to New Zealand from Germany in the 1970s, I encountered a theatrical scene that was very conventional, colonised by British expectations of repertory theatre and a Shakespearean kind of rhetorical performance, with received pronunciation – a kind of theatre that was not a specifically New Zealand theatre. There was some specifically national New Zealand theatre in content, but its form remained mainly locked into colonial models, and what I saw did not reflect what one would have been experiencing in Europe and the United States at the same time. In my view, New Zealand theatre served to represent middle-class domination and British colonisation.

Instead of claiming the moral high ground, Falkenberg catches himself in the trap of theatrical colonisation:

When I was asked to make theatre here, I tried to counterbalance this colonisation with another kind of colonisation by bringing in European, continental texts and physical theatre methods – starting with King Ubu, Dada, and Surrealist theatre – trying to emancipate the theatrical scene from this kind of British theatre and, through these 'antitheatrical' texts, to create a tabula rasa in order to be able to start anew.

(Falkenberg 2005: 39)

Recognising the impossibility of starting with a clean slate and resisting the impulse to make a theatre of denial, Falkenberg uses the rest of this slight polemic to outline his current thinking about a devising process that might preserve and, through a strategy of juxtapositioning, expose the ambivalence of making theatre in New Zealand:

Perhaps instead of conforming to a fixed script which is always in danger of being frozen in some other place, time, and ideology, it is better to look for identity through a provisional art, where texts and participants become the material of performance in a dialectical process. It may be, in the present situation, that there are no pure local identities any longer – if there ever were. A country that is built upon colonisation must be seen in the act of continually devising an identity for itself. How else to represent such acts if not by following the same provisional path?

(Falkenberg 2005: 40)

Falkenberg's Free Theatre productions are presented as acts of ongoing enquiry by company members, working with everything from classical texts to personal narratives, between theatre and film, song and dance, to create theatrical experiences that leave the audience with more questions than answers.[5] Seen as a kind of Turnerian social drama, these productions, at their best, eschew the comforts of the 'rite of return' and *communitas* in favour of an uneasy sort of liminoid open-endedness.[6] This approach to making challenging theatre about the essential problem of living here now has a number of obvious pitfalls. Leaving the audience to figure out what the performance has to do with them can lead them to grasp at straws, as happened during the recent production of *Distraction Camp*, a devised work that played with recycled playtexts and live reproductions of film scenes, much as the

Wooster Group does. Audiences loved it, for the most part, but the production was accused of excessive didacticism, even though the actors' most vehement proclamations explicitly engaged in, and linked, flagrant anti-Semitism with sexism in a way that should have made it hard for anyone to find prescriptive.

Most of the theatres in New Zealand seem to fall somewhere between these two extremes. The repertory (or community) theatre tradition here is a direct legacy of the colonial period, when settlers not only flocked to tours of British companies but also picked up playtexts and performed them for their own entertainment in community halls. Not so much has changed. In Christchurch, as I write this, while the Court Theatre is about to open Chekhov's *The Seagull* and the Free Theatre is about to open its revisioning of Marlowe's *Doctor Faustus*, we are also looking forward to seeing Sir Ian McKellen in *Wating for Godot* at the Isaac Theatre Royal, while just a few blocks away the Repertory Theatre is following up its sell-out season of *The Diary of Anne Frank* with *Journey's End*, both productions being labours of love for their many on- and off-stage participants and loved in return by the families, friends and acquaintances who make up the majority of the audience.

It's the same in other New Zealand provincial centres. Each has at least a quasi-professional company at its heart (for example, the Fortune in Dunedin, Centrepoint in Palmerston North). Each has a company or two operating at the fringe with a more radical – or at least provocative – premise. Each welcomes international touring companies with excitement at the opportunity to see stars live onstage and for a high culture experience but also a certain ambivalence about what it means to import such entertainments, the reflection of provincialism that is cast upon the audience and the reminder that it is far indeed from the Empire that produced such great plays.

This ambivalence toward the theatrical artifacts of British civilisation is at the root of the Pākehā New Zealander's theatrical experience, as Australian theatre scholars Helen Gilbert and Joanne Tompkins recognise in their groundbreaking book *Post-colonial Drama: Theory, Practice, Politics*: 'History is a particularly fraught issue for settler societies because of their ambivalent positioning in the imperial paradigm as both colonisers and colonised.' Postcolonial drama, they believe, must both reveal and deconstruct 'any continuing colonialist power structures and institutions' – an admittedly elusive objective whether one is queuing to see a knighted actor perform at the Isaac Royal Theatre or looking to a local, community theatre production of *Journey's End* (1992: 3, 113).

But for Gilbert and Tompkins, the theatre's role in confronting the legacy of colonisation is imperative: 'Post-colonial theatre's capacity to intervene publicly in social organisation and to critique political structures can be more extensive than the relatively isolated circumstances of written narrative and poetry' (3). Ironically, perhaps, given the central thrust of this chapter, one of the first stages in the journey from colony to country – if not the establishment of a national theatre – seems to be the theatricalisation of a national identity. For Gilbert and Tompkins: 'The multiply-coded representational systems of theatre offer a variety of opportunities for the recuperation of a post-colonial subjectivity which is not simply inscribed in written discourse but embodied through performance' (109).

Closer to home, University of Auckland academic Murray Edmond explicitly links theatre and nationalism in his personal history of the burgeoning experimental theatre movement during the 1970s and 1980s – if only to decry the slow coming of age of New Zealand theatre: 'Inasmuch as we wanted to produce a new theatre, we were part of a second coming of nationalism in the arts in New Zealand. The first coming of nationalism, in the 1930s and 1940s, had failed to achieve anything for the theatre when compared with, say, writing or painting or music' (Edmond 1996: 3).

Edmond stages the conflict between the colonial and the postcolonial as a struggle against the British theatrical tradition: 'For the experimental theatre, the new theatre had to destroy the old. But here, in New Zealand, the new theatre also had to be something of this place, of here' (23). There is, of course, something of a paradox in attempting to turn the theatre – an inherited art form and an instrument of colonisation – against itself as a way of breaking free of the colonial past. The problem of nation and theatre, separately and in relation to one another, is that there is no possibility of starting with a clean slate, even if one leaves Shakespeare and Shaw on the shelves. And yet, Edmond reports, this is what they tried to do: 'The self-created work was also the work of creating the self' (25).

Perhaps imagining that theatre and nation can be created by looking in a narrowly focused mirror becomes possible only on a small group of islands in the South Pacific – perhaps even more so in the relative isolation of the years when travel was expensive enough to mean that one was either here or there, and the distance was not mitigated by the Internet. Edmond and his collaborators sought to use theatrical practices as a way of finding out about New Zealand identity. Calling themselves the 'Town and Country Players,' they decided to 'take shows and workshops into the countryside, to schools and country halls, to be billeted with people, to set up a kind of cross-cultural contact with theatre as a means more than an end. The life of the country, its divisions as much as its unlikely coherencies, attracted us. The "theatre" would create a meeting' (Edmond 1996: 4). Devising theatre in and with rural communities in order to elicit a sense of national identity and communal purpose was not, in itself, so original by the 1980s, but at a time when New Zealand's identity was still largely bound up in its British exemplar, to assert that conversations over tea in a rural community hall might be a truer form of New Zealand theatre might have been no less radical in some ways that Boal's Theatre of the Oppressed was in its own context.

One of Edmond's critical observations is that the flames of nationalist fervour in 1970s New Zealand sparked the simultaneous founding both of conventional theatres such as the Court and of experimental theatre troupes, including, perhaps most famously, the Red Mole Theatre Ensemble by Sally Rodwell and Alan Brunton in Wellington in 1974 (Edmond 1996: 3–4). Red Mole quickly became notorious for the way they incorporated agit-prop and cabaret, clowning, masks, songs and dance, rejecting the conventions of British accents and vocal intonations – that is, the Britophilic pretensions common in New Zealand theatres of the time – in favour of their own regional accents and intonations, to produce satires on issues drawn from the local headlines. Their manifesto was driven by the exuberance of discovering themselves as New Zealanders, politically and theatrically:

1. to preserve romance;
2. to escape programmed behaviour by remaining erratic;
3. to preserve the unclear and inexplicit idioms of everyday speech;
4. to abhor the domination of any person over any other;
5. to expend energy.

(Edmond 1996: 304)

Red Mole were committed to discovering New Zealand onstage, touring throughout the country, gathering stories and company members peripatetically. They were social, theatrical and political magpies, interweaving local community-centred concerns, British popular performance traditions and European radical theatre theories and social philosophies. Yet, like Murray Edmond, Terry Snow, writing in 1978, essentialises New Zealand national identity as something that can be unearthed directly by turning away from the British past:

> It is this originality, this unwillingness to rely on received theatrical words or frameworks, combined with a happiness to embrace the first premises of popular theatre and the evolution of a recognisable local style stemming from the regular company, which has resulted in the unique contribution of Red Mole Enterprises to the New Zealand theatre scene.

(Snow 1978)

Ironically, Snow's essay appeared as the company was departing for foreign shores. It is telling that Red Mole's identification as a quintessentially New Zealand theatre company came about after they landed in New York for an extended residency, testing and consolidating their theatricalised version of a New Zealand identity as they travelled throughout the US and Europe throughout the 1980s. That is, to be seen as a New Zealand theatre company, by New Zealanders as well as by the international theatre community, Red Mole first had to be identified as such by non-New Zealanders first. Murray Edmond writes:

> Overseas, Red Mole found they could trade on their specific, local version of exoticism. In New York being from New Zealand had more currency than being from New York. From being alienated at home, they became ethnic overseas, but without losing their alienation. They doubled their value.[…] The doubling of value did not simply happen *over there*, it also happened *back there*. Red Mole in New York took on a mythic status at home. On their first return to New Zealand in 1980, Red Mole was able to sustain, even enhance their mythology. In New York they were wandering players from 'a small island in the South Pacific' – in New Zealand they are wandering heroes from the big, bad, seductive Apple. This logic worked well so long as their transient, 'on the road' status was maintained.

(Edmond 1996: 358)

In fact, Red Mole's international reputation meant that they were consistently cited by my New York colleagues as a great reason to move to New Zealand, and it was to my chagrin, as a geographically challenged American, that I discovered upon my arrival on the South Island the distance between Christchurch and Wellington put Red Mole essentially in another world. Fortunately, the other company most cited in New York, Pacific Underground, was based in Christchurch.[7] In fact, one of the first performances I saw here was a parody of *Bill and Ted's Excellent Adventure* in a community hall at the Youth Centre in Manchester Street. The room was full of Polynesian families, children racing around, adults chatting among themselves, laughing uproariously and talking back to the performers. It was the epitome of rough community theatre, indifferent to outsiders, and totally at home with its audience.

Founded in the early 1990s as a collective of musicians, writers and performers of Samoan extraction (including Oscar Kightley, Erolia Ifopo, Michelle Muagututi'a, Simon Small and Michael Hodgson), and as such situated outside the Māori–Pākehā binary, Pacific Underground are not so much troubled by the national identity question as with their own history of exclusion and oppression, having exchanged one island homeland for another, being neither Māori nor Pākehā, 'the Samoan predicament' (O'Donnell 2007a: 308). In his survey of Pacific theatre, David O'Donnell (2007a: 328) singles out Victor Rodger, who in plays such as *Ranterstantrum* and *My Name is Gary Cooper* confronts

> the discourses of racial separatism and strongly questions the popular perception of New Zealand as a racially tolerant society where white and Polynesian peoples live together in harmony. Rather than Aotearoa the 'bi-cultural paradise,' he depicts a post-colonial community fraught with divisions and misunderstandings. [...] There is real anger there, stemming from a collective 'mistaken identity,' a deep-seated inability among closed Palagi communities to recognise and to live alongside their Pacific neighbours.

Mixing satire with drama, pulling its theatricalities from television as well as sketch comedy and European realism, Pacific Underground's theatre work defines the wider New Zealand culture oppositionally. In contrast, many of the musicians, including Scribe and members of Fat Freddy's Drop, who have emerged from Pacific Underground's early performances have become iconic; their eclectic conflation of Pacific Island sounds and beats with hip hop, soul, R&B and funk has come to represent New Zealand's musical identity both nationally and internationally.

At base, the debate about New Zealand's identity – inside theatres and out – remains centred on and revolves around the Treaty of Waitangi, which is officially considered the nation's founding document. Despite its actual diversity, New Zealand culture continues to be defined by the colonial encounter between Māori and the first wave of British settlers, a bicultural drama that is played out between their descendents in a way that leaves many of us, unofficially at least, on the sidelines. It is the presence of Māori – their tribal histories and cultural practices – that distinguishes New Zealand from other postcolonial nations. After all, without the haka, the All Blacks would just be another rugby team representing a far corner of the former British Empire. This chapter's preoccupation with the relationship between the theatre and New Zealand's national identity necessarily culminates in a look at how the theatre, as a European art form, has been appropriated and developed on Māori terms in order to reflect and shape ideas about Māori cultural identity against the backdrop and oppressions of New Zealand's colonial history and its not quite postcolonial present.

Like the haka, Māori theatre seems to have come to dominate the international imagination about New Zealand's national identity, albeit in ways that are perhaps less about empowerment than about branding. Prominent New Zealand playwright, director and producer, and Māori theatre activist, Hone Kouka is probably best known for a series of plays he wrote in the 1990s. In his recent essay, 'Re-Colonising the Natives: The State of Contemporary Māori Theatre', Kouka (2007: 240) recalls being inspired in 1990 by *Whatungarongaro*, a play by the Māori theatre collective He Ara Hou, that he says, convinced him 'that this innovative Māori theatre really had no boundaries'. He goes on: 'For the first time in a piece of Māori theatre, I saw traditional Māori concepts and Western theatre practice integrate seamlessly and become a healthy theatrical hybrid.' An anonymous reviewer in the Te Pūtātara newsletter describes the production's innovations:

> It is not just the theme and the actors and the theatre that are Māori; but the kaupapa of the play, its internal structure and its presentation are totally Māori. Gone is the structure of the European play with its one, two or three acts and rigid adherence to linear European time. This play is presented as a single act, switching between future, past, distant past and present, with each event linked to the one before and to the one after, but in which the passage of time is coincidental. Time on this stage becomes Māori, telescoped into a single event. Linear time is relevant only in the passing of the seasons and of the generations.
>
> (15 November 1990)

Inspired by *Whatungarongaro*, Kouka interwove Ibsenian realism with aspects of Māori protocol in *Nga Tangata Toa* (1994) and in the plays that followed, establishing a model for Māori theatre in which the social issues facing Māori found expression in the interplay between European and Māori language and performance practices.

In his reflections on Māori theatre in twenty-first-century New Zealand, Kouka also looks to the development of Marae Theatre by Jim Moriarty and others as another way of negotiating theatrically with the impact of colonisation:

> This practice was entirely based around Māori tikanga and kawa (laws and rules), stipulating that, when audience members came into the theatre, they were treated as if they were entering a wharenui (traditional Māori meeting house), and therefore a Māori world. [...] I understood that Māori theatre can only be a hybrid, as in traditional Māori society the concept of a 'theatre' was foreign.
>
> (2007: 241)

In his essay, Kouka's primary concern is for the way the Māori theatrical voice – which seemed to prevail in the 1990s – has somehow again been submerged. He argues that Māori social and political issues are being ghettoised by the dominant, Pākehā, culture, once again suppressed or, as in this article, channelled by non-Māori writers:

> I read an article involving a cross section of New Zealand playwrights, in which a particular paragraph caught my attention. The Pākehā writer claimed that Māori and Pacific Island work was great currency for the international market place and these same Māori and Pacific Island stories and characters were very much considered as commodities. The words stung and reminded me of the land grab in New Zealand in the late nineteenth century or the self styled protectionism of anthropologists taking Māori taonga for our own good or the kehua of paternalism that still haunts us as a people today.
>
> (Kouka 2007: 238)

The theatre company that Hone Kouka directed for many years, Taki Rua, is still operating, along with his newer company, Tawata Productions, still generating new plays by and for Māori, provoking debates on contemporary social issues by experimenting with theatrical forms. Like the other theatre companies and artists considered in this chapter, the work done by Taki Rua sits successfully within its own community where a serious conversation about Māori social and political issues, as well as the nature of theatre in a postcolonial context, carries on largely out of the sight of the rest of us.

New Zealand does not have a national theatre, but it does have a National Drama School: Toi Whakaari. Toi Whakaari has evolved over the years, taking on a Māori name, for example, and intertwining aspects of Māori performance practice with more conventional forms of European theatre training. Students' work culminates in a series of devised solo performances, which presents them to the wider community simultaneously as individuals and a kind of representative group, the newest generation of New Zealand theatre artists. And then they scatter, intent on making careers within the limitations of the theatre, film and television industry here or they venture overseas. For a moment, though, in the graduating class, it is possible to catch a glimpse of what New Zealand looks like in the bodies and voices of its theatre aspirants, performing their diverse stories and identities in roughly the same structure, sharing the same stage, albeit not at the same time.

What might a national theatre in New Zealand look like, and what might such an institution accomplish that cannot be achieved by each of these groups on their own? Drawing together the threads of its own theatre history, a New Zealand national theatre might stage itself as a meeting place. Less concerned about the eyes of the world, and more curious about how theatrical ideas can be seen to shape as well as represent social ideas, a national theatre here might allow us to experience a more fluid sense of what it is to live together on this small, relatively isolated cluster of islands, to build a national identity that is not necessarily singular or unified but understood as composed of complementary, sometimes even divergent strands of historical movements, and to find new ways of weaving our individual performances together in art as in life.

Works cited

Anderson, B. [1983] (2006), *Imagined Communities: Reflections on the Origin and Spread of Nationalism*, London & New York: Verso.

Court Theatre (2010), *About Us*, Accessed 1 May 2010, from http://www.courttheatre.org.nz/index.cfm/1,9,html/About-Us.

Edmond, M. (1996), *Old Comrades of the Future: A History of Experimental Theatre in New Zealand, 1962–1982*, PhD Thesis, University of Auckland.

Falkenberg, P. (2005), 'Why Devise? Why Now? Why New Zealand?', in *Theatre Topics*, March, pp. 39–40.

Free Theatre Christchurch (2010), *History*, Accessed 1 May 2010, from http://www.freetheatre.org.nz/manifesto/his-index.shtml.

Gilbert, H., and Tompkins, J. (1992), *Post-colonial Drama: Theory, Practice, Politics*, London: Routledge.

Kouka, H. (2007), 'Re-Colonising the Natives: The State of Contemporary Māori Theatre', in M. Maufort and D. O'Donnell (eds.), *Performing Aotearoa: New Zealand Theatre and Drama in an Age of Transition*, Brussels: P.I.E. Peter Lang S.A., pp. 237–246.

Maufort, M., and O'Donnell, D. (eds.), (2007), *Performing Aotearoa: New Zealand Theatre and Drama in an Age of Transition*, Brussels: P.I.E. Peter Lang S.A.

O'Donnell, D. (2007a), 'Re-Claiming the 'Fob': The Immigrant Family in Samoan Drama', in M. Maufort and D. O'Donnell (eds.), *Performing Aotearoa: New Zealand Theatre and Drama in an Age of Transition*, Brussels: P.I.E. Peter Lang S.A., pp. 307–330.

—— (2007b), '"Whaddarya?" Questioning National Identity in New Zealand Drama', in M. Maufort and D. O'Donnell (eds.), *Performing Aotearoa: New Zealand Theatre and Drama in an Age of Transition*, Brussels: P.I.E. Peter Lang S.A., pp. 17–25.

Pacific Underground (2010), Accessed 1 May 2010, from http://www.myspace.com/pacificunderground.

Parker, G. (2008), *Actor Alone: Solo Performance in New Zealand*, PhD thesis, Theatre & Film Studies, University of Canterbury.

Royal Court Theatre (2010), *About Us*, Assessed 1 May 2010, from http://www.royalcourttheatre.com/about.asp?ArticleID=14.

Said, E. W. [1993] (1994), *Culture and Imperialism*, London: Vintage.

Snow, T. (1978), 'Red Mole', in *Art New Zealand*, Winter, Assessed 1 May 2010, from http://www.art-newzealand.com/Issues1to40/redmole.htm.

Te Pūtātara: A Newsletter for the Kumara Vine, 15 November 1990, Assessed 1 May 2010, from http://www.maorinews.com/putatara/puta_030.html.

Turner, V. (1982), *From Ritual to Theatre: The Human Seriousness of Play*, New York: PAJ Publications.

Notes

1 For an extended examination of the relationship between solo performance and national identity, including analyses of Mason and Thompson's work and impact on the development of New Zealand theatre, see George Parker's recent PhD thesis, *Actor Alone: Solo Performance in New Zealand* (Theatre & Film Studies, University of Canterbury, 2008). Academic studies of New Zealand theatre and performance are only now emerging, with *Performing Aotearoa: New Zealand Theatre and Drama in an Age of Transition*, a collection of essays edited by Marc Maufort and David O'Donnell (2007), the first major publication to survey the field with some depth. In particular, the essay by David O'Donnell, '"Whaddarya?" Questioning National Identity in New Zealand Drama,' addresses the history of New Zealand playwriting from the perspective of a New Zealand director and dramaturge who has been working at the heart of the issue for several decades.

2 See, for example, Edward Said's *Culture and Imperialism* (1994) and Benedict Anderson's discussion of 'Official Nationalism and Imperialism' in *Imagined Communities: Reflections on the Origin and Spread of Nationalism* (2006).

3 For example, the Mercury Theatre in Auckland and Downstage in Wellington.

4 This image is drawn, however awkwardly, from a well-established trope in NZ literature and film, especially *The Piano* (dir. Jane Campion, 1993).

5 For their manifesto and a list of productions, see the Free Theatre website: www.freetheatre. org.nz.

6 See Victor Turner, *From Ritual to Theatre: the Human Seriousness of Play* (1982).

7 See their website (http://www.myspace.com/pacificunderground) and also David O'Donnell's brief survey of their history and four key playtexts in 'Re-claiming the "Fob": The Immigrant Family in Samoan Drama' (2007a).

Chapter 7

Between Pride and Shame: A Dialogic Consideration of *Honour Bound* and *Reconciliation! What's the Story?* in Pursuit of an Australian National Identity

Rea Dennis

The turn of the century represents a period in which Australia generally has been preoccupied with the pursuit of a singular defining national identity narrative. This is linked to the ambivalent political environment nurtured under the four consecutive terms of liberal leadership with John Howard as Prime Minister. The collapse of the integrity of the multiculturalism and diversity narratives alongside a surge in border security narratives under Howard has exposed the fragility of the aspirations we have held for a coherent unifying national identity narrative. Of course, this has also been influenced by international events. As a young country we are locked into the search to find some fit between a global Australia and a local Australia. It is as if the need to confront the reality of our past has us stalled between invasion and settlement narratives and this, alongside the manipulation of what could be called the shame/pride narrative has characterised the past few decades in Australia. Since September 11, Australia's engagement in the War on Terror has led to a visceral exploitation of fragments of identity narrative. This has come in many forms, yet at its most basic appears as a question about the balance between the pursuit of our national security and the sanctity of our human rights. Prior to 9/11, the move towards reclaiming indigenous rights had bought into sharp relief the injustices of the past and a questioning of what it means to be Australian and what rights one must invoke in order to claim this identification.

Identity narratives are implicit in the stories we tell. Indeed narrative theory claims that stories are the most consistent and familiar way that we make sense of things that have happened and assist us to create how we'd like things to be. Bruner (1986) acknowledges the way in which public narrative enables us as a culture to be reflective and reflexive. Theatre provides a place in which societies can reflect. Giroux writes that such spaces must embrace a shifting ground of 'multiple and heterogeneous borders where different histories, languages, experiences and voices intermingle amid diverse relations of power and privilege' (1992: 32). It is this potential in theatre and performance that facilitates civic dialogue. Dialogue occurs when we are prepared to examine other positions, positions that might challenge and interrogate our own. That is, dialogue occurs when we are open to a more critical reception in the theatre, when a kind of transparency is present due to the exchange of stories, and who is telling and who is listening. In this chapter I set out to examine the faces of the contemporary national identity in Australia in the early twenty-first century through the dialogue surrounding two distinctly different theatre events.

Honour Bound (2006) had its world premiere at the Sydney Opera House on 2 August 2006. The creation of internationally renowned director Nigel Jamieson and Australian Dance Theatre choreographer Garry Stewart, *Honour Bound* is a culturally and artistically ambitious work that focuses on the experiences of Terry Hicks and his Australian-born son David Hicks. David was held by the US in Guantanamo Bay for four years without trial. The 70-minute long work features documentary material including Terry's personal testimony as a father, and also draws on letters, internal Pentagon papers and the accounts of former detainees. Attempting to raise questions about the sanctity of human rights, *Honour Bound* is said to integrate Jamieson's expertise in physical and aerial language and projected film and imagery. In a vastly different style, *Reconciliation! What's the Story?* (2002) was performed on 19 May 2002 at the Uniting Church Hall Merthyr Street, New Farm. Created in response to the Sorry Day[1] agenda, it was produced in collaboration with Brisbane Playback Theatre Company for my PhD research.[2] Also based on personal testimony, *Reconciliation! What's the Story?* (2002) sought to explore the social dimension of the Australian reconciliation debate through the everyday stories of audience members. The 90-minute performance featured over ten stories from the audience that were transformed by a team of actors and musicians into short theatrical works. Both *Honour Bound* and *Reconciliation! What's the Story?* are derivative of theatre methods based on personal narrative. It is not uncommon to see personal narrative extrapolated to illuminate a broader socio-cultural context. *Honour Bound* could be conceptualised as using Verbatim or Documentary Theatre as a point of departure for creative practice. *Reconciliation! What's the Story?* is more straightforward, based entirely on the interactive theatre method known as playback theatre. Playback theatre is a community-based performance form in which personal stories are told in a public performance, where this telling is juxtaposed with improvised dramatisations informed by the told story. I have written previously about how playback can offer a place of resistance and dialogue (Dennis 2007). When considered in terms of narrative, *Honour Bound* seeks to extrapolate one person's story into the broad international context of human rights as a way to examine the forces at play. Whereas *Reconciliation! What's the Story?* draws on many stories in a more anthropological or ethnographic kind of theatre event in which the broader context may come to be understood through reflection on a range of personal experiences and perspectives.

Both *Honour Bound* and *Reconciliation! What's the Story?* begin from a desire to explore the impact of government decisions on human rights. Both are produced during a period of ambiguity about what it means to be Australian; a period in which there had been a shift to a crude re-storying of the complexity of what it means to be Australian toward a simplistic values-based assessment of what qualifies as 'Australian' which is accomplished through the construction of some 'other', that which is 'Un-Australian'. It is not easy to write a context for this chapter. Australia is a small nation with a population of just 20 million people, and I am reluctant to add another simplistic construction to the pot of confusion. If I consider some of the research into what it means to be 'Australian', the popular position seems linked to sporting heroes on the one hand and iconic figures like 'diggers' on the other. Australian social scientists, Bruce Tranter and Jed Donoghue (2007) report that the contemporary Australian identity landscape is dominated by colonial and postcolonial figures rather than by ideas of nationhood. They nominate postcolonial historical figures such as the iconic digger from the ANZAC story and Post-Second World War immigrants as more influential in narratives of national identity and suggest that colonial figures like convicts, free settlers and bushrangers are far less important. Constructing the nation from a purely postcolonial position is limited. Tranter and Donoghue's study absents any trace of indigenous strands to the national narrative. The work of indigenous lawyer and academic Noel Pearson might provide some insights into this. For one thing, the contemporary reality for Australia's first people is that colonisation is not yet over. He states:

[T]here are people whose lands and societies are still at the frontier of exploitation [...] The traditional owner in Cape York does not want to wait another few years for her land to be alienated by mining development [...] The prospects for getting land back, when one's traditional lands are covered by sugar cane fields, becomes very dim.

(Pearson 2003)

In light of contemporary international dialogue, the status of first people, nationhood and indigenous rights are inhibited in Australia due in part to the way in which different jurisdictions such as Canada, the United States and New Zealand employ these terms in different ways. For example, 'Treaties in North American law, recognition of "first nations" in Canada and of "domestic dependent nationhood" in the United States [...] are primarily domestic concepts' (Furniss 2005: 31). Pearson (2003) suggests that the place of the indigenous voice is also confounded by the inadequate nature of the Western-originated understanding of nationhood. For aboriginal Australians there is a complex conception of 'nation' which poses a central dilemma in trying to construct nationhood in relation to pre-European Australia. The way in which the Western legal tradition describes 'nation states is artificial if applied to the Aboriginal relationship to land which is at the core of the indigenous domain' (Pearson 2003). This then represents an irreconcilable idea of nationhood and results in a stark alienation of Aboriginal people from such an Australian nation, and risks their ongoing erasure or omission from any national identity narrative.

This period equates to a time in which the Australian national narrative is in acute crisis in relation to the balance between local and global priorities – where issues of indigenous Australians rights have been overshadowed in the service of border security narratives and the aggressive undermining of the multicultural story. On the back of the 2000 Olympics, Australia was poised to ride the national pride wave well onto the beach of international belonging. The abhorrent treatment of asylum seekers in the Children Overboard scandal (Marr and Wilkinson 2003) put paid to the careful laundering achieved through the Olympic Opening Ceremony (OOC) in what appeared to be the accomplished re-storying of Australia into a nation that had finally arrived. Michael Cohen states that the OOC performances were designed to 'demonstrate that Australia was effectively "at home" in the world and they were arranged in a way to affirm that the Australian house was in (the right) order' (2006: 65). I use the concept of arrival intentionally. Australia has a long history of nation building based on arrivals. Ironically, the events of August 2001 contradict this narrative completely. I am referring here to the Australian government's refusal to allow the Scandinavian vessel, The Tampa, *to arrive*. The Tampa had entered Australian waters in desperate request of asylum. Not only did the government deny them refuge, they also made untrue public announcements, claiming the refugees were casting their children overboard (Marr and Wilkinson 2003). This incident drew a new wave of international attention to Australia, this time in relation to the political treatment of asylum seekers. In a spate of rapid narrative bites, Australia was soon recast as hostile and inhumane. If it wasn't for the shift of public attention to the centre of New York some two weeks later, there is no saying where this might have led. This period resulted in a shift away from local political issues like indigenous rights, towards an Australia in pursuit of a purely international identity. These rapid shifts of narrative positions inspired the 2002 performance *Reconciliation! What's the Story?* The 2005 production of *Honour Bound* was perhaps even more inspired by the aggressively constructed imperative of 'nation before human' narrative in the Australian story, seeking to question the way in which human rights become negotiable in times of national threat through the story of David Hicks. I begin this chapter from the position that both *Honour Bound* and *Reconciliation! What's the Story?* are about National Identity.

> *Behind the gates of Guatanamo. Into the world of David Hicks.*
>   (Sydney Stage, 2006, *Honour Bound* promotional material)

While the promotional material claims to be going somewhere other than here, *Honour Bound* could be said to be expressing the shadow past of the Australian invasion story. Jamieson is quoted as saying: 'My central ambition was to look at the Geneva Conventions, which were formed after World War II as a protection for people everywhere, and to explore through this particular story how quickly you fly into a bestial darkness, once you allow human beings to step beyond those frameworks [...] what it meant for us, as a people, to no longer respect human rights treaties' (London Evening Standard, 2007). Jamieson's claim is that he wants to reveal, to expose the wrongs of the past. Very similar sentiments are expressed in relation to the calls for a national apology to the aboriginal people and principle elements reinforcing the national narrative that could be conceived as the Shame/Pride Narrative in the Australian context.

The Shame/Pride Narrative is a complex phenomenon that characterises recent Australian history. In her 'Politics of Bad Feeling' essay, Sara Ahmed (2005) examines the way in which the Shame/Pride Narrative has its primary roots in the treatment of indigenous Australians during colonial invasion. In her detailed work analysing the Sorry books within the reconciliation culture, Ahmed has attempted to better construct the way in which living with shame is manifest in the Australian psyche. She cites Darwin to explain: 'under a keen sense of shame there is a strong desire for concealment' (2005: 75). Concealment or omission is a principle emerging theme in the dialogues surrounding the two performances. Inside the *Reconciliation! What's the Story?* performance a woman expresses her frustration about the absence of the indigenous history in her school room: 'Why weren't we taught this? Is it being taught today?' Later in the performance the actors set about creating a scene in response to Bruce's story. He has spoken about his cousin's recent work on the family tree and how this has uncovered a truth about his great grandmother – they had always believed that she was an exotic princess from Spain. But through the family tree research, they learn she is indigenous. He reflects on the culture of shame in the family that has led to them concealing this fact. He recalls his Dad's advice to him as a young man about not marrying his aboriginal girlfriend. It seems ironic he said, that we have this beloved grandmother who became a myth as an exotic Spanish Princess. The man, now in his fifties expressed his sadness that his father was not alive to know the truth.

The narrative of concealment also emerged through the discussion about omissions and errors in *Honour Bound*. In reaction to award winning Australia poet and theatre critic Alison Croggan's (2006) claim that

> Jamieson and this collaborators have simply done what is obvious. An admirable moral clarity informs every aesthetic decision, which gives the show a weight of honesty which can be difficult to find in the medium of theatre. This clear beginning, when dancers enter in their underwear and put on the familiar orange jumpsuit of detainees: this gesture, which reveals to us the artifice of theatre, permits its subsequent truthfulness.

The piece has been accused of having 'one glaring omission' (Phillips 2006). This discussion centres on the way in which *Honour Bound* fails to clearly establish how the Australian government, the Australian nation and ordinary Australians are complicit in Hick's detainment. Boyd (2006) and Williams (2006) point to this omission as a key weakness in the work. Boyd categorises the piece as quasi propaganda and is damning of the way in which 'it politely glossed over the Australian Government's complicity in the illegal and immoral incarceration of David Hick's.' This discussion about omission is frequently expressed in the broader social context in relation to politicians' behaviour.

This discussion opens the door for another dimension in the Shame/Pride Narrative, that of looking for someone to blame. In Phillips' (2006) critique of *Honour Bound*, he announces: there is a

> clear framing of Bush and Rumsfeld as the only bad guys in the political sphere. We don't follow up any of Howard or Ruddock's sustained demonisation of Hicks, and their continual undermining of his right to a fair trail. It is trust the USA all the way with our (Howard) government, and while the makers of the show can certainly assume that most of their audience will add this to the onstage action, the presence of this work so firmly in the mainstream makes this omission telling.

Williams (2006) also expresses his shock that Bush and Rumsfeld are presented as 'the only bad guys' and takes offence at the initial absence of acknowledgment by Jamieson of London's Tricycle Theatre (2004) production of the same name. Tricycle creates political tribunal performance and their *Honour Bound* has been described as the kind of play that Brecht would write if he were alive today. The Independent's theatre and dance commentator discusses the place of facts in Tricycle's work, in which 'everything depends on the power and truth of the narrative'; and where [t]he facts literally speak for themselves' (Whitaker 2004).

The culture of concealment and omission is perhaps characteristic of a country struggling to come to terms with its past. Diversity scholar, Mary Kalantzis suggests that omissions arise when they are linked to a narrative that is in counterpoint to what is desired. She calls it the second story; the one that is much harder to tell. She links this difficulty in telling to the way in which we remember; she says it is in the problem of 'how to remember things' that we wish to forget or deny (2001: 20). The difficult thing about telling the second story in the Australian context is that it requires us to admit fault or to be contrite. This difficulty manifest in the Australian context as the repeated and ongoing refusal by the Howard government to issue a formal apology to indigenous Australians.[3] The refusal to admit responsibility and to make amends is linked directly to what Ahmed calls 'the bind of shame'. She claims, shame is made real when others see us in light of our shameful behaviours. The witness is necessary. 'Sartre suggests that: "I am ashamed of myself as I appear to the other"' (cited in Ahmed 2005: 76). The principle way to avoid shame in the Australian context has been to blame the other.

The theme of Othering emerged in the dialogue of both performances. Erving Goffman (1986) first proposes his analysis of spoiled identity in relation to the construction of The Other through the reading and rejecting of difference. He examines how we use our reading of difference as deviant to justify an increase in social distance between self and the other. Berman links the compulsion to establish the one who is different from me as other to the rise of mirror manufacturing in the modern era which he aligns to the breakdown of 'Self/Other unity'. He suggests, '[n]ation-states, armies, self-portraits, perspectives, the collapse of magic – all these represent an increasing preoccupation with boundaries with sharp Self/Other distinctions' (1990: 49). This confusion is indeed manifest in Jamieson's Hicks. In his consideration of the national narratives that are vying to define what is Australian in the twenty-first century, Chris Wallace is unapologetic in his assessment of John Howard's focus on difference as *the* problem. He writes, 'multiculturalism, immigration, border security and indigenous policy all became sharp weapons in the government's re-election toolkit' (2007: 126). An Australian version of the US Culture Wars[4] saw Howard crusade against the so-called 'black armband view of history' (126); that perspective on Australian values 'that there was nothing in the national story worth celebrating' (Soutphommasane 2007: 136). Howard's election platforms progressively nurtured and exploited what Ahmed (2000) identifies as the contemporary fear of The Other and the way Howard used the discourse of stranger danger in direct contradiction to the long-term narrative pillar, multiculturalism, to destabilise it as a potentially coherent strand in the Australian national narrative.

The theme of the other as dangerous was present in the dialogue that emerged from the audience at *Reconciliation! What's the Story?* performance. During the performance a woman named Maria recounted one of her significant experiences as a child in which there was a mystery shrouding a certain railway station in the city. On trips to visit her grandmother, she would observe large groups of people paying particular attention to their personal space as the train prepared to arrive at Redfern; some, she said, seemed to be clinging to the walls of the carriages as the doors slid open. She told how she would try to steal a look around; to capture some glimpse of what might be on everybody minds, only to find nothing unusual (to her eyes) – people waiting for the train. As the doors slid closed and the train moved off, she remembered the feeling of the simultaneous out-breath of the strangers around her and would stare at her grandmother trying to understand. As an adult she has since come to understand more about the inner Sydney area of Redfern and its infamous indigenous population.[5] Yet, despite the notion of threat in Maria's story, the dialogue arising from *Reconciliation! What's the Story?* was more about difference than danger.

In an ironic inversion, in *Honour Bound* there is Hicks the white Australian-born boy who, despite his sameness, is constructed as the 'other' by the Australian government. As the commentaries of Williams and Phillips show, in choosing to gloss over the Howard government's accountability in Hicks' interment, Jamieson's piece effectively blames Bush. Yet there is a broader discussion about the other as dangerous that played out in relation to Hicks that cast him as the enemy. In part, the premise of *Honour Bound* appears to be concerned with the redemption of Hicks after he is blamed and then abandoned by the nation. Jamieson claims his purpose was to interrogate the way in which the Australia government acted to make Hicks the demon by nature of his religion. This mirrors the contemporary 'othering' of Muslims, and the automatic construction of a Muslim traveller as a terrorist. In a strange kind of twist, blame comes under an ambiguous kind of scrutiny in *Honour Bound*. Through the use of a range of theatrical techniques, the differentiation of 'us' and 'them' is continually blurred. Dancers wear identical jumpsuits, which obscures their differences. They switch between roles raising questions of identity: Who is Hicks? Who are the guards? Who is Muslim? Who is American? Who is the terrorist? There is no clear perpetrator. Similarly there is a kind of collision of these identities within the Hicks portrayed in the press – he is us and he is them. By way of humanising Hicks, Jamieson appears to take particular care to include background story of David Hicks before he joined Al Qaeda and ended up in Guantanamo Bay. Through a strategic placement of family photographs, David's childhood story is told. Through these simple and unsophisticated devices, Jamieson seeks to portray a flawed yet human David, someone a father loves and is proud of. It is likely Jamieson includes this material to build empathy amid his highly technical event. We meet a young version of Hicks, the Australian kid at home, a battler, flawed, a subsequent failure as a young adult searching for meaning in a range of jobs before finally choosing Islam. Yet in such a spectacular event, the placement of these personal artefacts has the appearance of trying to explain away Hicks' responsibility. In a manner similar to that of the immunity *Honour Bound* affords Howard, this sets up a kind of immunity for Hicks, a way to justify the road he has taken rather than to question what responsibility he has in it all. Perhaps both instances equate to some misguided elitism within the Australian narrative – that Australians are beyond blame. Or perhaps it is merely the outcome of an overt effort to avoid blaming Hicks. Williams (2006) offers an alternative reading, suggesting that Jamieson's inclusion of the personal material 'clearly' establishes Hicks' 'normality against his demonisation' and makes clear that 'what has happened to him could happen to any of us in this current climate'. We are them and they are us. This ambiguity also extended to content and form.

Gattenhof claims that a defining tenet of contemporary performance is the ubiquitous interaction of content and form where 'form equals content and content equals form' (2008: 153). In *Reconciliation! What's the Story?* the form derives from the oral tradition of storytelling and cultural performance (Fox 1994). The values implicit in the process are an indelible part of the performance experience. As an interactive theatre event participants are implicated in the content presented and the range of voices represented. It is by nature dialogic. By contrast, *Honour Bound* is 'performance innovation' (Gattenhof 2008, 154); where performance innovation equates to performance that 'informs us in a way that the medium never has before, through connections that redefine conceptual relationships in the craft' (Blumenthal cited in Gattenhof 2008: 154).

Much has been made of the physical/aerial/digital elements of Jamieson's production. Gattenhof who says the work was 'shatteringly good' cites Jamieson's endeavour as 'seeking to use a brutality of physical language in an attempt to function as an analogy to the psychological, emotional and physical turmoil' of Hicks (2008: 153). The choice to place a physical language at the centre tends to somewhat overwhelm the spectator. My own experience was to become distracted by the virtuosity of the bodies. Yet, such physicality is relevant in the experience of shame. Ahmed writes, 'the very physicality of shame – how it works in and through bodies – means that shame also involves the forming and reforming of bodily and social spaces, as bodies "turn away" from the others who witness the shame' (2005: 75). Stewart's dance language tends to be repetitive and draws overly on the more spectacular torture elements in the Hicks story. Boyd (2006) complains that it is didactic and 'unrelievably literal', suggesting that the choreographic language leaves little to the imagination. The scenography of metal frames and orange overalls are similarly overdrawn symbols in what Schechner (2002) has termed the theatre of terror. These elements undermine the scope of the dialogue and reinforce the feeling that something is being washed over or obscured. Perhaps it is the closeness of the form to the sensationalised TV broadcasting associated with the Hicks case and with reporting of the War on Terror generally. Spectacle is Nigel Jamieson's oeuvre with other memorable moments including *The Theft of Sita* (2000) and the *Tin Symphony* for the Opening Ceremony of the Sydney 2000 Olympics. By his own admission, Jamieson's (cited in an interview in the Evening Standard) motives were driven by sensationalism. He states:

> I'd seen a TV documentary about David's dad Terry, and the journey this working-class man had made from a northern Adelaide suburb to Afghanistan to find out what had happened to his son. I then had this image of a figure in an orange jumpsuit floating in a steel cage

and thought: 'I can make a piece of work out of that.' The tendency of the piece towards a sensationalist aesthetic reminiscent of television news broadcasts appeared to promote the kind of theatre of terror that Schechner (2002) criticises in news reportage after 9/11. This sensation is perhaps reinforced through the dominant use of media in the performance. The work of the artists Scott Otto (video) and Paul Charlier (sound) tends to skew the genre toward what Feldman has identified as flash image broadcasting – that broadcasting that uses the 'aggressive technologies of image making and image imposition' – which has the effect of destabilising the integrity of the work and shifts it beyond refracting or recording an event toward making the event intentionally 'political'.

(Feldman 2005: 205)

Drawn from a different theatre tradition, *Reconciliation! What's the Story?* is equally at risk of misrepresentation. The form relies on playback theatre; a simple or raw performance method based on audience stories and actor improvisations. In playback theatre, audience members provide the scripts. On the night approximately 60 people attended the performance and one by one, about 13 told stories. After each story the group of actors improvised a scene. The playback theatre aesthetic can tend to privilege the social practice of storytelling over the artistic practice of theatre making. Some audience members commented that while it was a thought-provoking event it was not high theatre. Perhaps interesting to note is that after the performance, more than half the audience remained in the auditorium in further discussion. The form itself is dialogic and in a way, the very local level of the theme and content of *Reconciliation! What's the Story?* replicated a kind of micro-society; a micro Australia. Story by story, improvisation by improvisation, the group engaged in a dialogue about saying sorry, the catholic concept of reconciliation, about keeping secrets, about needing to take sides, about standing up for your values and beliefs and about being prepared to consider the difference in yourself.

In addition to the performance content, *Reconciliation! What's the Story?* engaged people in difficult discussions. These could be perhaps considered a micro-version of the second story that Kalantzis (2001) claims are key to building coherence and congruence as a nation. Melanie[6] attended the night. A young woman in her thirties, she invited her mother to come with her. She cited her main purpose in bringing her mum was so she was not on her own, however she later spoke about the way in which the content of the performance led to a significant conversation between the two of them.

What was really great was that it generated discussion with my mother I'd never had before. I learned things about my mum I never knew and it led to a very deep discussion. I love her, and feel like she's my best friend, she's so gentle and caring and I didn't think she felt so strongly about things. She told me how she felt about the aboriginal stuff, 'they're not the only race or people whom suffered.' She's pretty angry that they (the aborigines) are still caught up in the anger. I haven't heard her talk about this stuff before, so I sat back and listened to her.

(Melanie, personal interview, 17 May 2002)

The way in which theatre enables a personal engagement is central to its dialogic potential. After the performance Craig and Luella (personal interview, 25 May 2002) found they too were immersed in a serious discussion about personal values and identity formation. It was just weeks before their first babies (twins) were expected. After the performance they found themselves in the midst of new territory openly and passionately discussing their values in relation to parenting. I include an excerpt of their conversation here. It arose in reference to a story told by a young woman during the performance, about her experience of prejudice in a corner store:

> Craig: That was the most powerful story that I found all night. It was about what I hold dear: it was about treating people with humanity [...] I look at everything with a 'parent hat' on now, that's a different perspective for me. I want my children to grow up with empathy and respect, and tolerance and understanding and ...
>
> Luella: and justice, and those sorts of things, and then we talked about – as parents, 'how do we make sure that our kids are respectful?'
>
> Craig: I would be horrified if my son treated someone like that, to me that would be the most horrific thing.
>
> (Craig and Luella personal interview, 25 May 2002)

Craig speaks about how the thought of his son mistreating someone would be 'horrific' to him. Luella questions the conditions needed to create respectful citizens. Both of them express concern about principle aspects of civil society not unique to Australia. The notion that lack of respect is 'horrific' is central to what Jamieson is seeking to say in *Honour Bound*. Perhaps this is why the narrative of national shame continues to underpin the dialogue about national identity in Australia. In the *Politics of Bad Feeling*, Sara Ahmed discusses the way in which the Sorry agenda sustains Australia's national shaming culture. She suggests that the Sorry books are a performance of shame and considers that the national shaming culture is a direct counterpoint to national pride. She equates national pride as achievable only through the act of recognising our brutal history. 'Such a narrative allows the national subject to identify with others, such that pride becomes an emotion that sticks the nation together, an ideal that requires the nation to pass through shame' (Ahmed 2005: 75). During *Reconciliation! What's the Story?* Hilary came to tell a story. In some respects she wants to talk about finding a place to express her pride. She came to the stage to tell about the ambivalence towards indigenous rights in her birth country. She begins her story by apologising, tentatively asking if her story can be included even though 'it's not about the Australian Aboriginals'. Hilary is a Cherokee and her story is about being forbidden to claim her ethnicity in the United States because of the rules associated with claiming indigenous identities in that country. The fact that she has been raised outside the Native American Indian tradition equates to having no rights. For her, Australia has been a place where she proudly expresses of her indigenous ancestry. The scene created from Hilary's story set the stage space up as two worlds: the United States and Australia. As the actors began to occupy these two worlds what is revealed is the sadness and guilt she felt in the United States juxtaposed to the pride and recognition she experiences in Australia.

It is ironic that throughout the dialogue arising from the two performances that a non-Australian born audience member expresses the principle feeling of pride. There is an uneasy relationship with patriotism in Australia. Linked in the past to sporting prowess and beach culture, more recently national pride has skewed towards a more American style patriotism. Political theorist, Tim Soutphommasane claims that Howard invoked this shift in direct opposition to former (Labour) Prime Minister Paul Keating's vision of Australia as one free from 'a British Imperial past' (Soutphommasane 2007: 135). John Howard's narrative position was based on the rediscovery of an 'authentic' Australian identity. The political rhetoric pursued the: Howard as hero, rescuing Australia 'from the muddle of multiculturalism' line; from a time in which we were 'obsessed with diversity' to a time to celebrate the 'enduring values of the national character' (Soutphommasane 2007: 134). However, in what could be seen as a modern day re-enactment, this kind of patriotism manifested most iconically, on the beach in the summer of 2005 where Sydney Morning Herald headlines called for Australians to *Stay off the Beach*. In a manifestation of national pride 'as racism and violence' by 'the mob of flag-waving chest-thumping Aussies at Cronulla who saw their actions simply as those of patriots trying to reclaim their way of life and national heritage' (Soutphommasane 207: 138). A distinctive image capturing the true national dilemma due to the erosion of multiculturalism, once again exposing Australian narrative identity as plural, conflicted and disaggregated.

Plural, conflicted and disaggregated could also be adjectives used to describe Hicks' identity. In *Honour Bound*, Hicks' story is a representation of the struggle for identification within Australia in the twenty-first century. This struggle is also present in the form of *Honour Bound*, reinforced in the creative decision to deploy the technically competent and identically-dressed dancers across a range of roles, which results in the dancers interchanging as prisoners and as interrogators: a deeply disturbing reality in our national history. Yet Jamieson's Hicks is a lost boy who does not belong, who is capable of criminal acts and of changing his cultural colours in order to fit in. This description could also be leveled at young Australia at the turn of the twenty-first century. Earlier I discussed the way in which the OOC sought to re-story Australia as having arrived. Indeed, since this spectacular event in 2000, Australia has invested in performance for export to Europe and Asia that seeks to reinforce a range of national narratives. Michael Cohen writes a provocative reflection on the way in which the OOC was used to reorganise and re-cast 'Australian nationhood on a global scale' (2006: 65) with an audience estimated at over 4 billion worldwide and 110,000 spectators present in the stadium. But national identity narratives cannot be re-written. This exploration of the dialogues inherent in and arising from *Honour Bound* and *Reconciliation! What's the Story?* shows an Australia searching for identification. It is revealing to consider the principle metaphors in *Honour Bound*: the cage (context) and the falling/flying body (subject) in relation to our preoccupation with defining a unifying identity. Perhaps the cage tells a story of a country bound by the past and lost in a present. The nations' past as a prison (steel cage) is centrally implicated in contemporary national distress with the free-falling body showing the way in which its people are suspended in limbo portraying the sense of dislocation and disorientation.

Epilogue: I am/Am I Australian(?)

Perhaps I, too, am like Hicks. I left Australia in search of some perspective on what has occurred in the years leading up to 9/11 and those following that culminated in a change of government and the history-making announcement by the incoming government that Australia apologises to the original inhabitants (Rudd 2008). Perhaps I, too, am like Hicks disoriented by the various national narratives and not feeling like I fit. I write this chapter from my home in Cardiff, Wales, yet do not feel like an expatriate in the way I always imagine Germaine Greer and Peter Carey did when I listened to their various defences in press interviews during my adolescence in the 1980s. Seven years ago, when I first left Australia, I was feeling feisty and ethically superior to that Australian majority who had so recently re-elected the conservative, pro-American, pro-war government of John Howard for a fourth term. In less than four months, Australia made headlines in the United Kingdom a number of times, and I am not referring to test cricket or to the Commonwealth Games. The riots on Cronulla beach in December 2005 were shocking and confronting. Along with many others, I was compelled to interrogate the way I viewed Australia. As I write, I remember a moment in my recent past where I felt something new in relation to Australia. Flying into the airspace above Brisbane, I felt myself 'home'. My reflection at the time was something like, 'Wow! Feel that Rea. That's it. Maybe that's the connection to place that aboriginal Australians feel. And feel that! You don't feel like you have to apologise for feeling connected to this land mass.' The kind of relief and grief that I felt in that moment is mine. I still take pleasure in the knowledge that I experienced that feeling, that I noticed my first ever feeling of the right to feel that I belonged to the land here. This chapter comes from the borders in my life that exist because I am a distanced citizen and despite my commitment to bringing a range of sources to bear on the discussion, I wish to acknowledge this very personal dimension. I construct this account in part from my own subjective lived experience accounts alongside theory, reflection and others' first person accounts in the way that Varela and Shear (1999) recommend. I also observe my tentativeness to write about Australia knowing that I embody a range of national identities that are in constant conflict.

Works cited

Ahmed, S. (2000), *Strange Encounters: Embodied Others in Post-coloniality*, London: Routledge.
_____ (2005), 'The Politics of Bad Feeling', *Australian Critical Race and Whiteness Studies Association Journal*, 1, pp. 72–85.

Berman, M. (1990), *Coming to Our Senses: Body and Spirit in the Hidden History of the West*, New York: Bantam Books.

Boyd, C. (2006), 'Comment', in Alison Croggan (ed.), *Honour Bound. Theatre Notes. Independent theatre review and commentary*, http://theatrenotes.blogspot.com/2006/09/honour-bound.html. Accessed 29 March 2010.

Bruner, J. (1986), *Actual Minds, Possible Worlds*, Cambridge, MA: Harvard University Press.

Cohen, M. (2006), 'Place and Dream-State: Spectacular representations of Nationhood at Stadium Australia', in Gay McAuley (ed.), *Unstable Ground: Performance and the Politics of Place*, Brussels: PIE Peter Lang, pp. 63–79.

Croggan, A. (2006), *Honour Bound. Theatre Notes. Independent theatre review and commentary*, http://theatrenotes.blogspot.com/2006/09/honour-bound.html. Accessed 29 March 2010.

Dennis, R. (2007), 'Inclusive Democracy: A Consideration of Playback Theatre with Refugee and Asylum Seekers', *Research in Drama Education*, 12: 3, pp. 355–370.

Feldman, A. (2005), 'On the Actuarial Gaze: From 9/11 to Abu Ghraib', *Cultural Studies*, 19: 2, pp. 203–226.

Furniss, E. (2005), 'Imagining the Frontier: Comparative Perspectives from Canada and Australia', in Deborah Bird and Richard Davis (eds.), *Dislocating the Frontier: Essaying the Mystique of the Outback*, Canberra: ANU e-press, pp. 23–46. http://epress.anu.edu.au/dtf/pdf/dtf_whole_book.pdf. Accessed 1 June 2010.

Gattenhof, S. (2008), 'Bound to Honour: The Detention of David Hicks as Performance', *Culture, Language and Representation*, 1, pp. 151–157, http://www.e-revistes.uji.es/index.php/clr/article/view/48/44. Accessed on 22 January 2010.

Giroux, H. A. (1992), *Border Crossings: Cultural Workers and the Politics of Education*, New York: Routledge.

Goffman, E. (1986), *Stigma: Notes on the Management of Spoiled Identity*, New York: Touchstone, Simon & Schuster: NY.

Kalantzis, M. (2001), 'Recognising Diversity', in M. Kalantzis and B. Cope (eds.), *Reconciliation, Multiculturalism, Identities: Difficult Dialogues, Sensible Solutions*, Victoria: Common Ground Publications, pp. 11–25.

London Evening Standard (2007), *Dance of the Detainee*, 13 November 2007, http://www.thisislondon.co.uk/arts/theatre/dance-of-the-detainee-6637854.html. Accessed 1 April 2010.

Marr, D., and Wilkinson, M. (2003), *Dark Victory*, Sydney: Allen and Unwin.

Pearson, N. (2003), 'Reconciliation: To Be or not to Be? Separate Aboriginal Nationhood or Aboriginal Self-determination and Self-government within the Australian Nation?' *Aboriginal Law Bulletin*, http://www.austlii.edu.au/au/journals/AboriginalLB/1993/12.html. Accessed 3 June 2010.

Phillips, R. (2006), 'A Passionate Exposure of the David Hicks Case, with One Glaring Omission', *World Wide Socialist Website*, 23 August, http://www.wsws.org/articles/2006/aug2006/hick-a23.shtml. Accessed 31 March 2010.

Rudd, K., on behalf of the Australian People (2008), *The Apology*. National Sorry Day Committee website, http://www.nsdc.org.au/home/index.php?option=com_content&view=section&layout=blog&id=8&Itemid=63&limitstart=9. Accessed 02 April 2010.

Schechner, R. (2002), 'Terrorism and Performance', in R. Schechner (ed.), *Performance Studies: An Introduction*, London, New York: Routledge, pp. 265–270.

Schultz, J. (2005), 'Colliding Worlds of People Unlike Us', *Griffith Review*, 8, pp. 7–11.

Soutphommasane, T. (2007), 'Surrendering Nationalism', *Griffith Review*, 16, pp. 133–140.

Sydney Stage (2006), 'Nigel Jamieson's Honour Bound', 28 July 2006, http://www.sydneystage. com.au/index.php?option=com_events&task=view_detail&agid=428&year=2006&month= 07&day=28&Itemid=34. Accessed 26 February 2010.

Tranter, B., and Donoghue, J. (2007), 'Colonial and Post-colonial Aspects of Australian Identity', *British Journal of Sociology*, 58: 2, pp. 165–183.

Varela, F., and Shear, J. (1999), 'First-person methodologies: What, why, how?' *Journal of Consciousness Studies*, 6: 2–3, pp. 1–14, http://www.imprint.co.uk/pdf/VFW_introduc.pdf. Accessed 24 January 2009.

Wallace, C. (2007), 'Libertarian Nation by Stealth', *Griffith Review*, 16, pp. 117–132.

Whitaker, R. (2004), 'Guantanamo – Honour Bound to Defend Freedom, Tricycle, London', *The Independent Theatre and Dance Website*, 30 May, http://www.independent.co.uk/arts-entertainment/theatre-dance/reviews/guantanamo–honor-bound-to-defendfreedom-tricycle-london-565362.html. Accessed 31 March 2010.

Williams, D. (2006), 'Comment', in Alison Croggan, (ed.), *Honour Bound. Theatre Notes. Independent theatre review and commentary.* http://theatrenotes.blogspot.com/2006/09/honour-bound.html. Accessed 29 March 2010.

Notes

1 Reconciliation Week and Sorry Day occur annually in May. In 2000 millions of Australians participated in a nationwide solidarity march for the rights and recognition of indigenous Australians. The surge in concern for refugees and asylum seekers in 2001 silenced the aboriginal agenda and Sorry Day 2001 was a low-key affair. After the September 11 attacks, Sorry Day 2002 was an opportunity to re-state the local issues alongside the global issues that are receiving attention in Australia.

2 The performance was aligned with my personal aspiration to contribute to the broader social dialogue on reconciliation in Brisbane. Local indigenous elders were consulted and advised us on various protocols to observe. This meant that the performance was promoted through indigenous agencies. Unfortunately, due to a death in the indigenous community that week, there were no aboriginal audience members.

3 This situation has since changed when on 13 February 2008, incoming Labour Prime Minister Kevin Rudd (2008) issued a formal apology to the Stolen Generation for the injustices they had endured under past government policies and practices. See a copy of the apology on the National Sorry Day Committee website at http://www.nsdc.org.au/home/index.php?option=com_content&view=section&layout=blog&id=8&Itemid=63&limitstart=9.

4 'In his 1991 book, *Culture Wars* (Basic Books), American sociologist James Davison Hunter identified a struggle between progressive and conservative values in America'; a battle which

'quickly became a political battlefield both in Oz and in the USA due to the direct and merciless readiness of political parties to exploit and amplify differences' (Schultz 2005).

5   See http://redfernoralhistory.org/ for an insight into the history of aboriginal life in Redfern.

6   Comments from Melanie, and later from Craig and Luella, were drawn from personal interviews conducted as part of my PhD research. Names have been changed as requested by informants.

Chapter 8

Under the Radar: Latin@/Hispanic Theatre in North Texas

Teresa Marrero

Introduction

The long-standing debate and lack of consensus about a singular, unifying theory as to terminology usage continues to mark discussions in the area of Hispanic/Latin@ studies in the United States. The hyphenated model of Mexican-American, Cuban-American, or the sweeping Hispanic versus Latin@ or even Chican@ (the @ eradicates the gender specificity of the Spanish a/o endings) point less to fragmented communities, but rather to ways in which the various ethnicities living in the United States, paradoxically, sometimes refuse and other times embrace the single identity marker ('I am not Hispanic, I am Mexican. I am Mexican but also Hispanic. I am both Latin@ and Chican@'). This opens options for ideological (re)alignments, thus enabling the possibilities to imagine one's self in multiple communities simultaneously. Because scholarship contributes to the production of collective identities (or lack thereof), as such, imagined academic communities establish spheres of intellectual influence that, in turn, bestow value upon the production of certain nations versus others, thus influencing not only self-perception but that of others. Part of this chapter discusses the type of relationship mainstream US theatre studies has had with Hispanic and Latin@ drama as a whole and the significance of this relationship for Hispanic and Latin@ identity.

The chapter will also discuss the more particular case of historic and popular identity formation in the state of Texas, using television series such as *Dallas*, and films such as *Giant* to draw the reader's attention to his/her own possible (pre)concepts about things 'Texan'. An overview of Hispanic stereotypes generated by the Hollywood film industry during the first and second halves of the twentieth century helps identify a shift from a positive (albeit glamorous and exotic) 'Latin bombshell/Latin Lover' to that of marginalised hoodlums in inner cities gangs after the 1960s.

The magnitude of influence produced by Hollywood surpasses that of any other, including that generated by live theatre. Thus, having to contend with mass-produced, stereotypes about Hispanics in film and television, bringing the issue down to the local level, Hispanic/Latino theatre artists are faced with challenges regarding their own viability as creators of cultural value. In spite of relative invisibility, there are five Hispanic/Latin@ theatre companies and various producing organisations currently active in the Dallas/Fort Worth Metroplex. A description of the facilities offers an idea of the type of spaces available for productions. My multiple roles as playwright and assistant director in two of the theatre companies included in this study have enriched my experience and appreciation of theatre workers in the non-profit sector. Thus a combination of the scholar and the working artist informs this chapter. I cull information from the results of an open-ended questionnaire I designed (see Addendum) and circulated among Dallas Hispanic/Latin@ theatre directors' views on issues such as language use (English, Spanish, or both), ethnic identity and casting, and perceptions of the visibility of their work to the general public.

Before we speak: Who are 'we'? Who am I?

Benedict Anderson's 1983 landmark and often-cited *Imagined Communities* proposed thinking of 'community' as a political entity, regardless of shared physical location or geographical boundaries. As Anderson puts it, a nation 'is imagined because the members of even the smallest nation will never know most of their fellow-members, meet them, or even hear of them, yet in the minds of each lives the image of their communion' (Anderson 1984: 6–7). Much scholarship has been generated since then. Within the area of Hispanic/Latin@ studies, Juan Flores states that the idea of 'imagined communities' lends itself well to the current conceptual terminology of Latino Studies because it helps to describe the 'national' experience of Latino diasporas in all its ambiguity, an important issue (Flores 2000: 213). Some scholars believe that the transnational nature of these diasporas have moved the topic beyond Anderson's initial concept into more complex systems of understanding communities-on-the-move on a global scale through the study of markets of consumption (Penaloza 1995: 83–94; 1994: 32–54, 2011: 131-161).[1]

Be that as it may, the point is that in the United States discussions of Hispanic/Latino cultural production (the arts, theatre, literature) are usually preambled with a sort of DNA string of citations regarding the preceding identity-politics debates within and about the various communities. Regardless of the topic at hand – be it theatre, performance, music, dance or any other cultural/artistic manifestation – we Latin@ scholars find ourselves in the Sisyphean task of perpetually attempting the impossible, that is, to fix definitions on the use of terms such as Hispanic versus Latin@, and positioning ourselves and our respective communities (i.e., often appearing to be 'speaking for'). Entering directly into a discussion of the specific artistic endeavour at hand thus becomes (necessarily?) cumbersome. This has been the case since I first entered the contested arena of Latin@ theatre in the United States in the early 1990s (Marero 1994: 102–120; 1991: 147–162; 1990: 147–153). The discourse of identity politics has become naturalised into the discussion of all Latin@/Hispanic cultural production. In contrast, scholars of US theatre do not feel the need to engage in a metaphysical discussion of what 'American' is prior to engaging in elaborations of the topic 'theatre'. This may change in the not-too-distant future when, according to demographic projections, 'the non-Hispanic white population will increase more slowly than other racial and ethnic groups; whites will become a minority (47%) by 2050' (U.S. Population Projections 2005–2050, 2008).

Upon reviewing the current theoretical discourse on Latin@/Hispanic identity politics, I see that, while the arguments have now been expanded to disciplines such as philosophy and to even that of geography, there continues to be a lack of uniformity or consensus as to which terminology is most suitable (Latin@ or Hispanic) (Garcia 2008; 2000, Garcia and de Greiff 2000, Arreola 2004). This impasse may, in itself, point to the futility of the endeavour. For instance, in the Dallas area there seems to be little identification (as there is, say, in other parts of Texas, such as San Antonio, or in California as a whole) with the term 'Chicano'. Academically, Chicano refers to Mexican/Americans who politically identify themselves and are aware of its socio-historical origins. Since my arrival in Texas from Southern California in 1992, I have heard the preferred terms to be Hispanic, Mexican-American or simply *Mexicanos* (with an 'x', my students insisted on this in a show of hands survey conducted on 30 March 2010, in my Latin American cinema class. Curiously out of 25, none identified themselves as 'Chican@' and only one as 'Latina'). This may be in keeping with the more politically conservative Texas social climate in contrast to the left-wing politics of the more radical California-based Chicano movement since its inception in the tumultuous 1960s. A noteworthy irony is that, even as I was writing this article, an executive from the Dallas area Spanish-language television mega network Univisión[2] wrote me an email requesting my professional advice: which might be the most appropriate way to name 'our' community, Hispanic or Latino? My suggestion was that if he were to conduct an audience survey, most respondents would identify as neither Hispanic nor Latino, but as Mexican, Cuban, Salvadorian, Argentinean (in other words, they would identify with their ethnicity of origin). The latest US census forms (2010 was a census year) have opted out of the dichotomous debate by offering further opportunities to self-identify racially and ethnically.[3]

On a more personal note, in recent years I refocused my participation in the cultural discourse as a creator of primary work rather than as a scholar. I redirected my attention towards creative writing, publishing short fiction and producing drama in Spanish (Marrero 2009).[4] I chose to work primarily with Spanish-language theatre, and not English. This contradicts the idea that those who work in Spanish do so because of lack of English fluency. It also goes against the commonly held notion that producing work for a majority (read: American English-language monolingual) audience ensures access into the 'mainstream'. For the most part, Hispanic/Latino theatre is valuable for the artists who produce work for the specific communities with whom they engage. My experience as Cubana/Latina/Hispanic has led me to choose that very possibility of cultural 'imagined communities', ones in which a person has the freedom to identify trans-culturally (and transnationally as in my case of identification with Argentina) and beyond linguistic colonisation (choosing Spanish rather than English for fiction and playwriting). While most of my research to date has dealt with US Latin@ theatre/performance, work generated in English (Marrero 2000), I now prefer to identify with an ever-growing population that frightens mainstream 'America'. That is, one that identifies itself culturally and linguistically with Spanish-speaking (with or without a hyphenated national identities) persons living in the United States, who were either born in Latin

America of various ethnicities, or born in the United States of a heritage linked ethnically to Latin America and who choose to retain Spanish as a significant if not dominant element in their lives, even while surrounded by an ever-growing wave of xenophobia.[5] As immigrants, we come to our new host country with or are inheritors of rich, non-Anglo cultural traditions which include theatre and literature.

World stages as seen through American scholarship: The nations that count

Because Hispanic/Latino theatre is created, produced, circulated and evaluated within the US cultural/educational scene, it is important to establish a certain context for its emergence into the 'sanctity' of critical discourse. Implicitly, imagined academic communities bestow value (i.e., privilege) to the production of some rather than others. As a representative sample, the publication history of one of the oldest and most prestigious journals in the United States, *The Drama Review* (known as *TDR*), provides a bird's eye view on the interests of US theatre scholars during the twentieth century.[6] Of note are evident absences, or, if one prefers a more politically neutral term, publication trends. The presences point towards the canonisation of some national theatres to the neglect of others. This is the case during the first two thirds of the twentieth century (up to the early 1970s) of American dramatic discourse, which has been predominantly preoccupied with establishing a creative and scholarly dialogue with Europe (read the United Kingdom, for obvious linguistic and historical connections, Greek classical drama, Germany for the work of Brecht, French theatre in its entirety including the Rumanian-born Ionesco, the Russian with Chekhov and Stanislavski, Italy with Pirandello, including an entire post-war issue rather belatedly in Spring 1964, topics related to the task of the actor and acting methodologies, Americans Arthur Miller, Tennessee Williams, Harold Pinter, Joseph Chaikin, etc.) to the exclusion of other European nations such as Spain, Portugal and Eastern Europe (except Poland whose Jerzy Grotowski comes to light in 1964 through Richard Schechner), as well as, frankly, the rest of the world! Latin American theatre, which boasts a rich history since the early 1900s in countries such as Argentina, Mexico, Peru and Cuba, does not appear on the radar until recently.

Spanish Golden Age theatre (fifteenth to seventeenth centuries) can hardly be considered an upstart on the world stage, with writers such as Pedro Calderón de la Barca, Miguel de Cervantes and Lope de Vega. However, one finds the first inclusion of an article on Spanish theatre in *TDR* to be on the Spanish Drama of the Golden Age, published in the late 1950s (Parker 1959: 42–59). It is not until the following year, that another Spaniard, Alfonso Sastre, makes an appearance as a subject of interest (Pronko 1960: 102–110, Decoster 1960: 121–132). A translation of a Calderón de la Barca play is published – a full year later (Calderón de la Barca and Muir 1963: 157–217). His work does not again appear as the subject of inquiry until three years later, in 1966. By 1971 the specificity of this 'other' theatre begins to appear more frequently, with articles dedicated to both Indian and Moscow theatre (Houghton 1971: 117–126, Withey 1971: 127–134). In the same year Maxine Klein is the first to publish a study on the theatre of the ancient Mayan (Klein 1971: 269–276), Japanese Kabuki and Indian ritual reappear in a subsequent issue (Pronko 1971: 409–430, McNamara 1971: 431–445).

Ironically, a review of a Chicano theatre piece makes its way into this American journal before anything Latin American. In October 1973 the journal publishes the first performance review of the landmark Chicano Teatro Campesino *La Carpa de los Rasquachis (The Tent of the Underdogs)*, performed at the Chelsea Theater Center, at The Brooklyn Academy of Music in New York City on 19 April 1972 (Brokow 1973: 267–268). As is common knowledge, Teatro Campesino emerged in solidarity with the Delano, California United Farm Workers' strike in 1965. Six years after their appearance in the US national, political arena, Chicano theatre finds recognition in a mainstream American theatre journal. In 1974 John W. Brokow, then professor at the University of Texas, Austin, reviews in Mexico City, three of Teatro Campesino's most well-known *actos: Dos peones* [sic] *por patroncito* (*Dos peones para el patroncito/Two Workers for the Bossman), Los Venditos* [sic] *(Los vendidos/Those Who Have Sold Out)*, and *El soldado razo* [sic] translated by Brokow as *Soldier of Race* (Brokow 1974: 108–111) whereas Chicano theatre scholar Jorge Huerta correctly translates it as *Soldado razo/Buck Private*.

Jorge Huerta's first book, *Chicano Theater: Themes and Forms* (Huerta 1982: 243–265) has an extensive bibliographic reference. It is of interest to note that while ethnic-specific journals such as *Revista Chicano-Riqueña, Caracol*, and *Latin American Theatre Review* figure prominently and often, thus bearing the brunt of exposing Chicano theatre to a specialised readership, mainstream US theatre journals such as *The Drama Review* and *Educational Theatre Journal* are also present, even if sporadically.

By the end of 1970 other neglected world cultural production, the African ritual and drama, is honoured in *TDR* with a single article dedicated to the entire continent (Graham-White 1970: 339–349), as if saying 'African' were equal to saying 'German' or 'French'. To my knowledge European cultural production is usually referred to individually by national or ethnic identity, and not as a continental conglomerate, such as 'African' (as of 2012, there are 47 countries in continental Africa and 53 if off-shore islands are included), 'Latin American' (20 countries) or 'Latino/Hispanic' (according to the US Census in 2008 15.4 per cent of the overall 304,059,724 US residents belong to this category).[7] It is misleading to ontologically present, and therefore perceive, these areas with an all-encompassing unity ('identity as nation') they do not possess.

In spite of a long and rich Latin American theatre/performance history, pre-Colombian[8] to the present, particularly in modern day Mexico, Peru, Argentina and Cuba, little of this cultural production is known or valued in the United States in spite of geographic proximity or large immigrant populations. A special issue of *Theatre Journal* dedicated to Latin American Theatre and published in 2004, engages mainstream US theatre studies with that of its neighbours to the south. Edited by Spanish-speaking Latin American theatre specialist Jean Graham-Jones, I had the opportunity of participating in the Forum (Marrero 2004: 254–256) as did the much respected and now Emeritus professor Jorge Huerta, who declared: 'It is no great revelation to say outright that our theatre departments remain Eurocentric in their curriculum and programming. Faculty, students, and guest directors select a play from the canon and that canon does not usually include Latino/a or Latin American plays in translation' (Huerta 2004: 472). In the same issue, the title of Adam Versényi's contribution to the Forum makes a powerful statement: 'You mean, there is a theatre in Latin America? This is the typical question I would receive a little over twenty years ago when I began to talk about my burgeoning interest in Latin American theatre' (Versényi 2004: 445). The following statement is worth repeating: the absence of knowledge or recognition of the United States' closest neighbours is astonishing, given not only the geographic proximity, but the migratory and thus cultural penetration. Graham-Jones puts it this way:

> **Latin America does not terminate at the U.S.–Mexican border;** thus although I'm cognizant of the attendant complications when including the U.S. Latino/a communities in a discussion of Latin American theatre, **the cultural network is such that I consider any arbitrary separation counter to the purposes of this reflection.** Otherwise, how can we take into account the larger networks navigated by such U.S.-based playwrights as Guillermo Reyes (born in Chile but raised in the United States and the author of plays about Chilean history as well as specifically U.S. identities) or Ariel Dorfman (born in Argentina, raised in New York City and Santiago, Chile, now a professor at Duke, and author of English-language plays whose subject matter is frequently authoritarian Latin America)? (Bold mine)
>
> (Graham-Jones 2006: 209–215)

Graham-Jones's statement highlighted above clearly concurs with my observations that to exscind Latin@ theatre from the Latin American is to create artificial national boundaries that do not exist. Likewise, to compartmentalise Latin@ theatre away from mainstream US production is to deny the most evident of facts: that we live transnational lives within a specific geographic location. According to the Pew Hispanic Research Center, 'nearly one in five Americans (19%) will be an immigrant in 2050, compared with one in eight (12%) in 2005' (www.pewhispanic.org).[9]

While the complexity of Latin American immigrant identities is an important issue to consider within the construct of 'imagined communitites', not all cases of Hispanic/Latino presence are the result of migration, as is the case of the Mexican communities in the present-day US territory belonging to Mexico prior to 1848. The states of New Mexico, Arizona, and California, parts of Nevada, Utah and Colorado were settled by Spaniards and Mexicans; however, Texas distinguishes itself within this group.

Texas: The lone star nation, popular imagination and Hispanic Hollywood

Texas is the only present-day state of the Union that can boast of formerly being a sovereign nation. After the Texas Revolution (October 1835–April 1836) the Texas Declaration of Independence from Mexico was adopted by the Republic of Texas at the Convention of 1836 at Washington-on-the-Brazos on 2 March 1836. Known as the Republic of Texas between

1836 and 1846, the territory of the present-day state of Texas was won in the Treaties of Velasco, with land from the Mexican states of Coahuila and Tejas. Mexico never recognised the loss of its territory, and this contested boundary has given way to constant discord between the two countries. The Texas flag, its identity as the Lone Star state, the outline of its geographic borders, the state flower (the blue bonnet), the state animal (the armadillo), and many other signifiers today abundantly remind Texans and non-Texans alike of where they stand. This proliferation of small nation markers creates a consciousness of nationalism that stands significantly *different* from that of other states in the union. These markers also attempt to establish a strong non-Mexican identity. It is as if by establishing its independence from Mexico and from the United States, Texas nationalism projects its image as uniquely standing alone and different ('the lone star state').

Because of its geographic immensity (696,241 sq. km), all things Texan appear in the (global?) popular imaginary as hyper real, expansive, big. Possible contributors to this notion are popular media such as television and film. *Dallas,* the prime-time television soap opera that originally ran from 1978 to 1991 on CBS and marketed in reruns worldwide, is a case at hand. Texas meant big sky and wealth from the oil and cattle-ranching industries. This show recycles stereotypical notions of what it means to be 'Texan' (read 'larger than life'). Hollywood cinema is an important transnational presence that may contribute to popular notions of 'Texas', as in the case of James Dean's last film, *Giant* (1956), directed by George Stevens and starring Elizabeth Taylor and Rock Hudson. As in *Dallas,* it repeats the themes of open spaces, wealthy oil barons and cattle ranching as synonymous with Texas. However, a subplot deals with a struggle between Anglos and Hispanics (led by Sal Mineo). 'Though the sprawling and leisurely picture dotes on its Anglos stars and themes, its ending which involves intermarriage, is significant [...] it makes clear, via the resultant offspring, that the future will ... have to be shared' (Hadley-García 1993: 151). The Anglo dominance goes unquestioned. Hadley-García suggests, in his landmark book *Hispanic Hollywood, the Latins in Motion Pictures* (1993), that the Mexican presence begins to demand visibility and attention at the symbolic level. Together with another popular television series, *Gunsmoke* (on the radio between 1952 and 1955, then on television between 1955 and 1975), an image of Texas and the 'West' was created in the popular imagination which read the 'frontier' as expansive, wild, larger than life and, curiously enough, eminently non-Mexican, considering that Texas was formerly a Mexican state, and that in 2008, 36.5 per cent of its residents are of Mexican origin (www.quickfacts.census.gov/qfd/states/48000.html).

The Mexican/Hispanic/Latino presence as a negative stereotype in Hollywood film appears as a post-Second World War phenomenon, one which Hispanics battle against today as artists and as general audiences. Presented with negative stereotypes, Hispanic consumers of popular Hollywood films struggle to see their communities represented in a positive way. *Hispanic Hollywood* clearly divides Hispanic presence according to the decades. From the advent of silent films through the 1920s, 1930s, 1940s and even into the 1950s, the Latin presence was esteemed as glamorous and desirable in a positive, highly marketable sense. Mexican female leading women such as Dolores del Río and Lupe Vélez were two of the most successful

Mexican actresses ever to cross over into Hollywood (Hadley-García 1993: 27). Followed by the Dominican María Montez, Mexicans Lupita Tovar, and Kati Jurado, they appealed to mainstream American audiences with their talent and beauty. This is ironic within the context of Texas secondary school educational policies in the 1960s as charted by Dallas' Cara Mía Theatre's 2009–2010 production *Crystal City, 1969*. Mexican/American students staged a walkout protesting racial prejudices, which, among others, barred Mexican female students from being elected as 'most-attractive', and as cheerleaders. Obviously, notions of 'beauty' respond to factors other than aesthetic, much to the chagrin of Kantian arguments. Judgments of beauty, in this context, are not 'disinterested', 'universal', nor 'necessary'.

By the 1940s, American film audiences had developed a taste for seeing films on location, allowing a gentle and benign penetration of the 'foreign' into the US imaginary, thus extending across the North/South continental axis the notion of a trans-America. The images of modern cities of Buenos Aires, Havana, Mexico City and Rio de Janerio paralleled those of New York in film and postcards, becoming household words of positive stature in the United States.

By the 1960s this perspective shifted towards representations of urban gangs (*Young Savages* and *West Side Story* both from 1961). Both set Puerto Ricans as poor ethnic minorities in New York's Spanish Harlem. From the 1960s to date, Hispanics in both film and theatre often complain of being offered limited, secondary roles as urban Mexican, Puerto Rican and Cuban gang members, secretaries, cheap manual labourers, and maids. Hollywood blockbuster films cast Hispanics as Mafioso Italians (Cuban Andy García in *The Godfather Part III*, 1990), or vice versa (Al Pacino as Cuban in *Scarface*, 1983, and *Carlito's Way*, 1993). The film industry mass-produces identity in ways no other media can. Residues of stereotypes created in one sector of cultural production bleed onto others, thus affecting general perceptions of Latin@s/Hispanics (in general and in the United States). As such, we are faced with a double task: that of deconstructing simplistic identities created for us by others, and of constructing creative, complex ones for and by ourselves and our various communities, albeit on a modest scale. David Lozano, Artistic Director of Cara Mía Theatre, comments below on the challenges of typecasting even ten years ago in Dallas, when the opportunities for 'brown' actors were limited.

Under the Texas sky: Theatre in North Texas

In 2009 Sarah Hart published an article for Theater Communications Group entitled 'Under the Texas Sky, A Flourishing Theatre Scene Thrives for Recognition Deep in the Heart of Texas' (Hart 2009) that provoked me to reflect: if the general Dallas theatre is striving for recognition, what can be said about the Hispanic/Latin@ scene? Inadvertently, she provided the present study with its title. In her article she drew an accurate sketch of the theatrical scene in the 'Big D' (the economic and cultural hub of North Texas). In brief, Hart offered a few relevant observations on theatre in a geographic area of roughly 9286 square miles

(24100 sq. km) composed of Dallas to the east, Arlington in the middle, Fort Worth to the west and Denton to the north. She states:

> The Dallas Chamber of Commerce estimates that there are 36 professional and community theatres in the city alone – yet Dallas still resists a reputation as a theatre town. [...] the business of competing with Texas priorities and ducking Texas stereotypes takes a toll on dramatic life here. It's hard, artists say, to be heard above the din – above sports and local politics and presidential flybys. Editors don't treat theatre as newsworthy bemoan others, citing the lack of press coverage in both cities [Dallas and Fort Worth] as a debilitating evil. Funding options (Texas ranks dead last in state support of the arts) fall prey to theatre's below-the-radar status when businesses or corporations want to affix their monikers to big things – for theatres are not big places that provide big exposure.
>
> (Hart 2009)

If these were the conditions with which mainstream (read Anglo) theatre has to toil, that is, 'below-the-radar status', what could be said of Hispanic/Latino theatre? Several of Hart's concerns also show up in the artist responses to my questionnaire. Lack of adequate newspaper critics/coverage is singled out as an eminent factor. Of importance is the implied notion that what Hispanics/Latin@s create has questionable relevance to mainstream consumers/audiences (thus being seen as economically not viable by business communities) relates directly to notions elaborated earlier in this chapter. Relative notions of worth stereotypically projected onto nations deemed inferior on the world stage questions the legitimacy and value of their contributions. (With all due respect to the Bard, why is it necessary to appeal to Shakespeare in order to gain legitimacy? Why not Calderón de la Barca, or Lope de Vega or the excellent work of Ecuador's Malayerba, or Peru's Yuyachkani, or Argentina's Mauricio Kartún, or Cuban-American María Irene Fornés, or that of Teatro Campesino?) All of the above share high aesthetic standards and thematic universality.

Dwindling economic resources in a depressed economy affects all, but some, such as David Lozano, question the ratio of distribution of city/state economic resources:

> I don't believe foundations, public agencies or even individual donors are funding Latino arts groups with a percentage of funds that matches the percentage of Latinos in the Dallas population ... Latinos make up approximately 35% of the population, but are Latino organisations receiving 35% of the funding? Are the theatre critics bilingual?
>
> (questionnaire)

In spite of above-stated setbacks, Hart comes to the conclusion that 'intensely loyal and intrepid art-seekers find when they do venture beneath the hullabaloo that there is a healthy range of theatre artists prepared to offer everything from large-scale, energy-infused musicals to edgy, unpredictable uncategoriseable performance' (Hart 2009). With regards to Latino Theatre, Hart states that 1985

> [s]aw the advent of the Latino company Teatro Dallas. Founder Cora Cardona worked against the grain to convince her community that a theatre of its own was essential – but she prevailed, eventually instituting a theatre that embraced the many heritages encompassed by Latino-American culture. … Dallas's brightest, if not steadiest, young theatre groups, including such special-interest companies as Echo Theatre (which performs works by women), Bucket Productions (which devotes itself to classics) and Teatro offspring Cara Mía.
>
> (Hart 2009)

All good intentions aside, at the time of Hart's publication, there were not two but five working Hispanic/Latin@ theatre groups in the Dallas/Fort Worth area. This ironically points to our relative invisibility, even to those well-intentioned, Anglo critics/researchers.

Working Latino theatre in the Dallas/Fort Worth areas: A real presence

At the time of writing this chapter, there are five Hispanic/Latin@ theatre groups operating in the Dallas/Fort Worth areas: Teatro Dallas, founded in 1985 by Jeff Hurst and Mexican actor/director Cora Cardona; Cara Mía Theatre Company, founded in 1996 by Eliberto Gonzalez and Adelina Anthony, is an offshoot of Teatro Dallas, and David Lozano (Chicano) is its present artistic director; Centro Cultural Argentino Grupo de Teatro, currently called 'Dr. Pedro Paez', founded in 1996 and is currently directed by Lilia Goldin; Teatro Flor Candela was founded in 2006 and directed by Patricia Urbina (Mexico); and Cambalache Teatro en Español, an offshoot of Centro Cultural Argentino, was founded in 2008 and is directed by Beatriz Mariel (Argentina). I (Cuba) was a founding member of Teatro Flor Candela and worked with this predominantly Mexican, Spanish-language group for its first year; I worked between 2008 and 2010 with Cambalache Teatro en Español, a predominantly Argentinean group, as playwright, and co-director. In 2009 and 2010 we produced my dramatised monologue set in Buenos Aires (adapted from a series of short stories published by Corregidor in Argentina), entitled La familia (Marrero 2009).

As far as venues are concerned, there are numerous cultural centres with fully equipped theatre spaces which belong to the city of Dallas and one belongs to Fort Worth. Two have Hispanic/Latin@ identity markers and function as producing organisations where local Latin@ companies may present their work: the Latino Cultural Center established in 2003, in the expensive district of downtown Dallas, and Artes de la Rosa, established in 1999, housed at the Rose Marine Theatre (formerly a movie house, now a theatre) in North Fort Worth (the so-called 'Northside Hispanic district' is demographically lower-income Mexican, Mexican-American, or Mexicano). The Rose Marine Theater, home of Artes de la Rosa, has the longest relationship with its community. It is listed on the National Register of Historic places. Of the five companies mentioned above, only Teatro Flor Candela is based in Fort Worth, Dallas's smaller sister city, although the company often presents programming for Hispanic children (mask-making and clown shows based on Mexican or Latin American mythologies) and acting workshops for adults based on anthropological, physical theatre at the Latino Cultural Center and at the Dallas Public Library, among others. All of the theatre companies and cultural centres operate as non-profit organisations, some receive funding from the City of Dallas Office of Cultural Affairs (OCA), and not all have received public funding.[10] Only Teatro Dallas operates its own theatrical space, although certain major events do take place at the Latino Cultural Center rather than at Teatro Dallas's home stage.

According to its website, the Dallas OCA is custodian of 19 city-owned cultural facilities of which five are operated directly, referring to them as 'cultural centers'. The Latino Cultural Center, among other publicly sponsored organisations, suffered budget cuts in 2009 due to the economic recession. With the largest annual operating budget of approximately 500,000 dollars, Dallas City Manager Mary Suhm stated in a 2009 interview with *Dallas Morning News* journalist Mercedes Olivera that 'all city departments, except for police, fire and code compliance, were facing 25–30 percent cuts [...] I know it's particularly hard for arts programs because arts funding is so difficult right now' (Olivera 2009). While there were no program cancellations for events already on the calendar for 2009–2010, Rose Marine Theatre executive Adam Adolfo, however did mention (see comments below) programming cancellations for 2009. Nevertheless, the following Dallas area Cultural Centers are listed as production venues of Hispanic/Latin@ theatrical events:

- Latino Cultural Center, downtown Dallas: the newest (2003), largest and most prestigious of the Latino producing organisations. 'Designed by world-known Mexico City modernist architect Ricardo Legorreta, it is a colourful, unique structure near the Dallas downtown area. It is a 27,000 square-foot, 300 seat theatre, a multi-purpose room, an art gallery, and sculpture courtyards that are widely used by local, regional, and international artists [...] The Mission of the Latino Cultural Center is to serve as a regional catalyst for the preservation, development, and promotion of Latino and Hispanic arts and culture' (www.dallasculture.org). While the LCC is available to all Latino performing groups, most prefer to stage their works first in smaller venues. Teatro Dallas presents some of the annual International Hispanic Theatre Festival here.
- Bath House Cultural Center, White Rock Lake, Dallas: 'Welcomes visual and a performing artists from an array of backgrounds. The historic, Art Deco style Bath House houses a 116-seat black-box theatre, three gallery spaces, the White Rock Lake Museum, and a number of multipurpose spaces' (www.dallasculture.org). This space is often used by smaller Latino theatre groups including Cambalache Teatro, Teatro Flor Candela, Cara Mia and Centro Cultural Argentino. My Spanish-language play *La familia* produced by Cambalache Teatro was staged there in November 2009.

- Ice House Cultural Center (1997)/Oak Cliff Cultural Center (2011): After being closed for renovations the Center reopened in with a new name. It provides community-based arts and cultural programming for the North Oak Cliff and West Dallas communities. These communities are traditionally Mexican and Mexican-American. The area is considered less than prestigious. Like the Bath House in White Rock Lake, it serves smaller theatre companies which were not linked directly with the Oak Cliff communities (www. dallasculture.org).
- South Dallas Cultural Center, South Dallas (1982): is a 24,000 square-foot multipurpose facility dedicated to the African American community. This centre is rarely used by the Latino performing groups, although the SDCC sometimes co-sponsors Afro-Latino music and dance events (www.dallasculture.org).

Not part of the Dallas Office of Cultural Affairs, but part of the city budget is the Dallas Public Library, directed by Miriam Rodríguez (Cuban). The library has a state of the art auditorium in the semi-round often used by Hispanic companies for performances and readings.[11] Thus it is a valuable venue of production, even though the space is not equipped with a proscenium stage.

In Fort Worth, the Rose Marine Theatre (a registered Texas historical site with a 254 seating capacity) houses its Hispanic project called Artes de la Rosa. According to its executive director, Adam Adolfo, '2009 saw the cancellation of theatre events. 2010–2011 will see the return of theatre to Artes de la Rosa … among shows (not yet publicly announced) will include a Cuban inspired *Cat on a Hot Tin Roof*, a Spanglish production of *The Vagina Monologues*, a theatre piece using modern Spanish poetry and the stage musical adaptation of the book, *Kiss of the Spider Woman*' (questionnaire). The relatively conservative programming is part of a plan to overcome 'the stigma' of getting general audiences 'interested in Spanish theatre' (all comments by Adolfo from the questionnaire). Thus the programming of 'mainstream' works is flavoured in generic Hispanic sauce in order to appeal to a wider audience. The implicit argument is that, first, the Hispanic community is not sufficient in terms of numbers to support its own theatre, and that, secondly, Hispanic themes need to be Anglicised in order to become palatable to an audience that is perceived as theatre supporting.

The questionnaire: If there are so many venues and theatre companies, why the relative invisibility?

For this chapter, I electronically circulated an open-ended English-Spanish questionnaire with 12 areas, plus one for 'Further Comments' at the end (see Addendum). Respondents were, in no particular order: Cora Cardona (Teatro Dallas), David Lozano (Cara Mía), Adam Adolfo (Rose Marine Theatre), Beatriz Mariel (Cambalache Teatro), and informally via the telephone, Lilia Goldin (Centro Argentino). The position of Manager for the Latino Cultural Center is presently vacant, thus my figures were culled from public websites from the City of Dallas. My contact for Flor Candela Teatro was unable to respond in a timely manner. By participating in the questionnaire, the respondents authorised me to quote their responses for this chapter.

It is fitting that pioneer Cora Cardona, founder and director of Teatro Dallas, celebrating its 25th anniversary in 2010, should lead the pack with her observations. Cora Cardona is a Mexico City-trained professional actress and director, whose primary language is Spanish. It is significant that, while I wrote the questionnaire bilingually, Cardona responded in Spanish (David Lozano of Cara Mía in English, Adam Adolfo for Rose Marine in English, Beatriz Mariel in Spanish, Lilia Goldin responded via telephone in Spanish, and had Flor Candela responded in a timely fashion in order to be included, Mexican actress/director Patricia Urbina would have responded in Spanish).

Cardona is a highly influential figure in the city, having a leading role in developing the Latino Cultural Center. Her role in the presence of a Hispanic/Latin@ theatre today in Dallas cannot be overestimated. In fact, most of the finely trained Latin@ actors in the area owe a debt to Cardona, for it was she who has seen it as her mission since 1985 to train Latin@ actors in a place where no academic or professional training program existed. Teatro Dallas identifies itself as a professional, non-profit theatre (all artists are paid), with an annual operating budget of 220,000 dollars, by far the largest of all Latino theatres in the city. They receive funding from the City of Dallas, the Office of Cultural Affairs, the Texas Commission on the Arts, sometimes the National Endowment for the Arts, various foundations, corporations and individual donors. It employs two full-time persons, four-to-eight per administrative project and between four and twelve per artistic project. The theatre has its own space (Teatro Dallas: 1331 Record Crossing Road, Dallas, TX 75235) with an expandable capacity between 45 to 65 seats; the space is available for rent when not in production. There is a fully functioning website. Their mission statement on the website states that 'Teatro Dallas is a non-profit professional theatrical institution dedicated to the presentation of all styles of theatre that reflect the varied cultural experiences of the Latino communities, through the works by both classical and contemporary Latino playwrights' (www.teatrodallas.org). Curiously, the Spanish language version of the mission statement varies the identity markers a bit: 'Teatro Dallas es un teatro latinoamericano en el área de Dallas/Fort Worth dedicado a la presentación de dramaturgos estadounidenses de origen latino e iberoaméricanos clásicos y contemporáneos' (www.teatrodallas.org). In Spanish, the identity is established as Latin American, with the contribution of US Latin@ and Iberoamerican classical and contemporary playwrights. With the exception of the International Theater Festival, which brings in works in not only Spanish, but a variety of languages, and its program of 'Domingos Fantásticos' (whereby plays are in Spanish), generally, Teatro Dallas produces plays in English. They do so, according to Cardona in the questionnaire, because (all translations are mine) 'this way we can reach a wider multicultural audience in order to better promote Spanish-language theatre' ('así abarcamos a un público más multicultural para difundir mejor el teatro de habla hispana') (questionnaire). While not mentioned in the questionnaire, city funding may have something to do with the language option, as public funding prioritises servicing the general population.[12] For example, librettos in English are offered to the audience during the multilingual International Theatre Festival. During the 2009 regular season they produced *Orinoco* by Mexican Emilio Carballido (a popular play on the Teatro Dallas repertory), *Blue Beach* (*Playa Azul*) by Mexican Víctor Hugo Rascón Banda (another favourite author at TD), and *La máscara que hablaba* (part of Domingos Fantásticos) by Alfredo Cardona Peña.

On the issue of visibility, Cardona believes that producing works in English as the *lingua franca* integrates them into the city's international ethnic communities. She believes that of utmost importance is having more theatre newspaper critics, because on the whole, they are 'disappearing' (questionnaire). She sees the urgent need to have professional Spanish-language theatre critics because, while the English-speaking ones can appreciate the artistic values of a Hispanic production, they are unable to elaborate on the cultural aspects of a work. The lack of media (newspaper, television and radio) coverage of theatre events is seen as problematic by not only Cardona, but by Beatriz Mariel of Cambalache, and David Lozano of Cara Mía.

An offspring of Teatro Dallas, Cara Mía Theatre, a non-profit theatre company, was founded in 1996 by Eliberto Gonzalez and Adelina Anthony, and is now headed by Chicano artist David Lozano. Its mission is

> [t]o broaden appreciation and understanding of Chicano and Latino culture through theatre, literature and educational programs […] filled a void in the Dallas arts community by becoming the first Dallas theatre to focus on the Mexican-American experience. Cara Mía assured Mexican-American audiences that their bilingual and bicultural experiences were represented regularly on Dallas stages.
>
> (www.caramiatheatre.com)

Cara Mía has presented works by established Chican@ playwrights, such as Cherrié Moraga (*Shadow of a Man*), by their own artistic ensemble (*To DIE:GO, in Leaves, Cholos y Chulas*) by David Lozano and Jeffry Farrell (*Nuestra Pastorela*), by Rodney Garza (*El Chuco y La Che*). *Crystal City, 1969*, their 2009–2010 project by David Lozano and Raúl Treviño, was based on historical research of a Mexican-American student walkout of the Texas Crystal City High School due to racial discrimination (at the time Spanish was forbidden in the classroom, students were spanked, slapped in the face, humiliated, Mexican-American students were prohibited from joining varsity sports, cheerleading, from being elected as most popular or homecoming court). The play, based on testimonials of those who actually participated and are presently successful members[13] of the community was a very powerful statement. Using ethnographic interview processes, the play, as well as the video documentation posted on the Cara Mía website (www.caramiatheatre.com), engages the community in an empowering (re)presentation of Mexican-American students as active participants in the American Civil Rights movement. Clearly, the production choices of Teatro Dallas and Cara Mía address the needs of different generations.

Lozano trained with Teatro Dallas for five years, under Cora Cardona, who has been extremely active in the task of training multi-ethnic actors in the craft of acting, staging, lighting and stage management. After a stint as apprentice under Cardona, Lozano began to attend University as well as work as Artistic Director of Cara Mía. Then, Lozano had an awakening. His testimony merits the lengthy quote:

Toward the end of my time at UTD [University of Dallas], professor Thomas Riccio asked me to create an original piece with actors from my company [Cara Mía]. He visited a rehearsal in which half of our group was from Mexico, the other half was Chicano. Up to that point, all of our Chicano teatro was made in English with some Spanish. Very little Spanish. At Teatro Dallas, plays were 90% in English. Well, Tomas saw a rehearsal and pulled me aside afterward and said, 'Don't you realise that you're asking Mexican actors to improvise and create scenes in English? It's not their language! They should be improvising in their maternal language, Mexican and Chicano actors performing in English show me a colonised theatre. Be true to the voice of your actors!' From then on, I changed my approach to making theatre. It was going to be bilingual. It was not important if Spanish speakers didn't understand some of the English and if the English speakers didn't understand the Spanish. That is how we live in Texas, not understanding what the others are saying.

(questionnaire)

Cara Mía presently produces work about 70 per cent in English and 30 per cent in Spanish. They do not attempt to 'neutralise' spoken accents. Defiantly, Lozano asks: 'Do we need to conform to an English-speaking culture? At Cara Mía, the answer is a resounding 'NO!' (questionnaire). A member for several years of the experimental Our Endeavors Theatre Collective (1997–2005), Lozano became further trained in the collective creation processes, although his first collaborative experiences developed working with Jeffry Farrell. Also, and possibly as significant, according to him, the Collective began showcasing the talents of Latino actors, such as that of Christina Vela, John Flores, Frank Mendez and himself (all originally of Teatro Dallas) and 'other companies began to cast us in ... roles not stereotypically asking for Latinos'. He played one of the leads in *Two Gentlemen of Verona*. David Lugo, a Mexican actor who had a major role, had the following observation: 'Who would have ever imagined seeing two Mexican actors playing principals on the stage at the Dallas Shakespeare Festival?' (questionnaire). Now, almost ten years later, Lozano recognises his good fortune to have gotten into the aperture for actors 'with brown skin' in Dallas.

The chapter closes now with companies whose work is clearly defined by the community they are part of, the Centro Argentino de Dallas has been producing work for the

Spanish-speaking Argentine community since 1996. They do not receive city funding and mostly produce entertaining light comedies. Beatriz Mariel, founder and director of Cambalache[14] Teatro en Español, was director for Centro Argentino productions since its beginnings. A self-taught-artist in her seventies, Mariel, in my opinion, is one of the most talented directors in Dallas. In 2008 she, as well as core members of the company, Maru Mariel, Daniel Chamero, and Nora Moreno, amicably broke away from the Centro Argentino in order to go devolve into more challenging works. Other stable present members include Cristián Muñóz (Chile), Fernando Garrido (Argentina) and myself (Cuba). Casting for two of the female roles in the 2009 production went to Jessica Rodríguez (Mexico) and Karla Silva (Mexico). None of the members are paid; thus far, the operating budget of the group is approximately 5000 dollars per annum. Rehearsals generally take place for six months prior to producing one play per year. In 2008 they successfully produced *El método Gronhölm* by the Catalan Jordi Galcerán Ferrer at the MAC Kitchen Dog Theater in Dallas. I worked with the group on this production as assistant to the director, and patiently awaited the opportunity to present them with my monologues, *La familia*, adapted from a series of eight stories published in book, *Entre la Argentina y Cuba: Cuentos nómadas de viajes y tangos* (*Between Argentina and Cuba: Nomad Stories of Travels and Tangos* [Marrero 2009]). They are eight characters written in Spanish with Argentinean voices. This is the only group in Dallas who could pull it off, and they did. In October–November 2009 the play made its debut in an alternative artist space and later at the Bath House Cultural Center. In 2010, the company will have re-staged their two best-sellers, Galcerán's play and mine.

As participant in the co-direction in Cambalache's productions, I can attest to at least one of the issues brought up by Cardona, Lozano and Mariel: the almost total neglect by the newspaper critics (both in Spanish-language newspapers and in Anglo newspapers). *La familia* played to audiences through word of mouth, flyers, free radio promotional spots, Hispanic email lists and Hispanic-interest websites. The audience was a cultural mix. This is not an easy play, and the characters are presented to the audience so that the audience participates in constructing the relationships between them. True to the characters' voices, the language reflects Argentinean argot not easily understood outside of this community. Not advertised as specifically 'Argentinean', comments from the audience during the Q&A afterward mentioned that the universal interest of the theme trumped any specific national markers. Although the core members of Cambalache are all bilingual in English and Spanish, we insist on doing theatre in Spanish. For Mariel the purpose is to preserve and promote the richness of the language (questionnaire). For me, it is simply a matter of acknowledging the loss that occurs in translation. Why mutilate my characters to speak in a language foreign to them, when there is a Dallas theatrical community who can deliver the story and a Spanish-speaking community who can enjoy the reception in the original language? Cambalache Teatro en Español offers Spanish-speaking communities an opportunity for thematic variety in a predominantly Mexican area.

Spanish-language theatre has even less visibility than most who are larger, older, and work in English or bilingually. Nevertheless, we continue to fill the modest spaces with a culturally sophisticated Hispanic population in the Dallas area (Mexicans, Argentineans, Cubans, Mexican-Americans, Colombians, Chileans, etc.) with quality work, coming full circle to the notion of imagined communities. While some of us are theatre professionals, others aficionados, and yet others stride the line between scholars and creators, we share the same vision: to do theatre for and by ourselves in language communities that belongs to the growing majority of the US population.

Addendum

Cuestionario ABIERTO / Open-ended questionnaire

(Circulated February 2010)

Created by TERESA MARRERO

(california_cuban@yahoo.com/ Teresa Marrero on FB)

Associate Professor of Latin American Literature, Theatre and Film, Creative Writer, University of North Texas

Favor de responder cuanto antes (o para el 5 de marzo a más tardar).
Please respond as soon as possible (or before March 5 at the latest).

Hola Teatreros:

¡Gracias por participar en esta encuesta! Estoy escribiendo un ensayo académico dedicado al teatro mundial. Mi ensayo incluye información demográfica y cultural relacionada a la presencia del teatro hispano/latino/chicano en el Metroplex. El título de mi artículo es, aproximadamente 'Por debajo del radar: el teatro latino/a en el Norte de Texas'. Alude a la relativa invisibilidad de nuestro teatro en relación a la gran actividad teatral que desempe–a nuestra comunidad. Mi meta es añadir un granito de arena hacia ponernos en el mapa cultural internacional. Con su participación en esta encuesta usted me autoriza para citarle en el ensayo. ¡Muchas gracias!

Estoy entrevistando dirigentes de teatros hispanos y directores de teatro:

I am working on an article dedicated to Theatre worldwide. My article deals with demographic and cultural data related to the presence of Hispanic/Latino/Chicano theatre in the DFW area. The title of my article is 'Under the Radar: Latina/o Theatre in North Texas'. The title alludes to the relative invisibility of our theatre community in relationship to its numerous activities. My goal is to add a small grain of sand towards placing us on the international cultural map. By participating in this survey you authorise me to quote you in my article.

I am focusing on interviewing Hispanic/Latino directors of cultural institutions and theatre directors.

FAVOR DE RESPONDER EN LOS ESPACIOS ENTRE LAS PREGUNTAS. LUEGO GUáDELO COMO .DOC Y DEVUéLVAMELO ADJUNTO A: **california_cuban@yahoo. com** *TEMA: ENCUESTA TEATRO. GRACIAS.*

PLEASE INSERT YOUR RESPONSES IN THE SPACES PROVIDED BELOW. SAVE IT AS A .DOC AND RETURN IT TO ME AT: california_cuban@yahoo.com SUBJECT: TEATRO SURVEY. Thank you.

IDENTIDAD/ IDENTITY

1. Por favor escriba su nombre, el nombre de su teatro/grupo, y su puesto dentro de la organización.

Please state your name, the name of your group, and your affiliation with the organisation.

2. Por favor diga la fecha de inicio de su grupo de teatro actual. Por favor declare si trabajó con otra(s) entidades teatrales antes.

Please state your present theatre group's date of birth. Please clarify if you belonged to other theatre group(s) prior to one with whom you are presently involved.

ESTATUS/ STATUS

1. ¿Cuál es su estatus legal (organización sin fines de lucro, teatro profesional, etc.)? ¿Cuán fácil/ difícil le resultó lograr este estátus legal?

   What is your status (non-profit, professional, etc.)? And, how easy/difficult did you find it to attain this legal status?

2. ¿Si su grupo tiene estatus de organización sin fines de lucro, cuáles son sus fuentes primarias de apoyo-ingresos y cuál es, aproximadamente, su presupuesto anual de operaciones?

   If your organisation is non-profit, what are your primary sources of support/income, and what is approximately, your annual operating budget?

3. ¿Cuántas personas emplea a tiempo complete y a tiempo parcial su organización?

   How many persons are employed full/ part time by your organisation?

ESPACIO/ SPACE

Su grupo de teatro tiene su propio espacio/ teatro: Sí _____ No _____
Your theatre group has its own theatre/space: Yes _____ No _____
Si no, entonces ¿dónde presenta sus obras?
If no, then where do you present your work?

LENGUA/LANGUAGE:

Su grupo hace puestas en escena en ¿cuál idioma y por qué?
Your group presents works in which language and why.

PÚBLICO/AUDIENCE

Su público es (la población de habla hispana, la población bilingüe, adultos, niňos, la población en general, etc.).
Your target audience is (Spanish speakers, bilingual, adults, children, the general audience, etc.):

RECENT WORKS or PROJECTS / OBRAS o PROYECTOS RECIENTES

¿Cuáles son algunas de sus obras más recientes (digamos el año 2009) y qué tipo de publicidad (medios de comunicación) tuvo para promoverlas?
What are some of your more recent works (say in 2009) and what sort of publicity (media) did you employ for promotion?

PERCEPCIÓN/ PERCEPTION

¿Cree que el teatro hispano/latino/ chicano en el Metroplex tiene la visibilidad que merece? ¿Por qué sí o no?
Do you believe that Hispanic/Latino/Chicano theatre in the Metroplex has the visibility it deserves? Why or why not?

¿SITIO WEB? WEBSITE?

Su organización/teatro tiene un sitio web. Sí _____ No _____
Your organisation/theatre has a website? Yes _____ No _____

OTROS COMENTARIOS / OTHER COMMENTS

Por favor, aproveche este espacio para añadir cualquier comentario que desee relacionado al tema. Please feel free to use this space to make any comments related to the topic at hand.

Works cited

Anderson, B. (1984), *Imagined Communities: Reflections on the Origin and Spread of Nationalism*, London: Verso, pp. 6–7.

Arreola, D. D. (2004), *Hispanic Spaces, Latino Places*, Austin: University of Texas Press.

Brokow, John W. (1973), 'Theatre in Review', *Educational Theatre Journal*, 25:3 (October), pp. 367–368.

—— (1974), 'Theatre in Review', *Educational Theatre Journal*, 26:1 (March), pp. 108–111.

Calderón de la Barca, P. and Muir, K. (1963), 'A House with Two Doors Is Difficult to Guard: (Casa con dos puertas mala es de guardar)', *The Tulane Drama Review*, 8:1 (autumn), pp. 157–217.

Decoster, C. C. (1960), 'Alfonso Sastre', *The Tulane Drama Review*, 5:2 (December), pp. 121–132.

Flores, J. (2000), *From Bomba to Hip-Hop*, New York: Columbia University Press, p. 213.

Garcia, J. J. E. (2000), *Hispanic/Latino Identity, a Philosophical Perspective*, Oxford and Massachusetts: Blackwell Publishers.

—— (2008), *Latinos in America, Philosophy and Social Identity*, Oxford, Massachusetts and Victoria: Blackwell Publishers.

Garcia, J. J. E., and de Greiff, P. (2000), *Hispanic/Latino Ethnicity, Race, and Rights*, London: Routledge.

Graham-Jones, J. (2006), 'Latin American(ist) Theatre History: Bridging the Divides', *Theatre Survey*, 47:2, pp. 209–215.

Graham-White, A. (1970), 'Ritual and Drama in Africa', *Educational Theatre Journal*, 22:4 (December), pp. 339–349.

Hadley-García, G. (1993), *Hispanics in Hollywood, the Latins in Motion Pictures*, New York: Carol Publishing Group, p. 151.

Hart, S. (2009), 'Under the Texas Sky, a Flourishing Theatre Scene Strives for Recognition Deep in the Heart of Texas', *Theatre Communications Group* , 17 March, ww.tcg.org/publications/at/2003/texas.cfm. Accessed 2 June 2009.

Houghton, N. (1971), 'Moscow Theatre 1935 and 1970: This Is Where I Came In', *Educational Theatre Journal*, 23:2 (May), pp. 117–126.

Huerta, J. (1982), *Chicano Theatre: Themes and Forms*, Ypsilanti, Michigan: Bilingual Press/Editorial Bilingüe, pp. 242–265.

—— (2004), 'Theatre as a Wild Weed', *Theatre Journal*, 56:3 (October), pp. 454–456.

Klein, M. (1971), 'Theatre of the Ancient Maya', *Educational Theatre Journal*, 23:3 (October), pp. 269–276.

Marrero, T. (1990), 'The 1989 Hispanic Playwrights Project at South Coast Repertory Theater: the Issues, the Plays, the Contest', *Gestos, Teoría y Práctica del Teatro Hispánico*, 5:9 (April), pp. 147–153.

——— (1991), 'Chicano/Latino Self-Representation in Theater and Performance Art: A Current View', *Gestos, Teoría y Práctica del Teatro Hispánico*, 6:11 (April), pp. 147–162.

——— (1994), 'Performance Art, Public Art: The Politics of Site', in Diana Taylor & Juan Villegas (eds), *Negotiating Performance: Gender, Sexuality, & Theatricality in Latin/o America*, Durham: Duke University Press, pp. 102–120.

——— (2000), *Out of the Fringe, Latino/a Theatre and Performance*, New York: Theatre Communications Group.

——— (2004), 'Theatre as a Wild Weed', *Theatre Journal*, 56:3 (October), pp. 454–456.

——— (2009), *Entre la Argentina y Cuba: cuentos nómadas de viajes y tangos*, Buenos Aires: Corregidor.

——— *La familia*, unpublished play script.

McNamara, B. (1971), 'The Indian Medicine Show', *Educational Theatre Journal*, 23:4 (December), pp. 431–445.

Olivera, M. (2009), 'Dallas' Latino Cultural Center Gets Stung With Budget Cuts', Saturday 4 July, http://www.dallasnews.com/sharedcontent/dws/dn/localnews/columnists/molivera/stories. Accessed 1 May 2010.

Parker, A. A. (1959), 'The Approach to the Spanish Drama of the Golden Age', *The Tulane Drama Review*, 4:1 (September), pp. 42–59.

Penaloza, L. (1994), 'Atravesando Fronteras/Border Crossings: A Critical Ethnographic Exploration of the Consumer Acculturation of Mexican Immigrants', *Journal of Consumer Research*, 21:1 (June), pp. 32–54.

——— (1995), 'Immigrant Consumers: Marketing and Public Policy Considerations in the Global Economy', *Journal of Public Policy & Marketing*, 14:1, pp. 83–94.

Penaloza, L. and Cavazos Arroyos, J. (2011), 'Here, There, and Beyond: Remittances in Transnational Family Consumption', *Teoría y Praxis*, 10, pp. 131–161.

Pronko, L. C. (1960), 'Alfonso Sastre', *The Tulane Drama Review*, 5:2 (December), pp. 102–110.

——— (1971), 'Learning Kabuki: The Training Program of the National Theatre of Japan', *Educational Theatre Journal*, 23:4 (December), pp. 409–430.

US Census 2010 Form (2010), Printed by the U.S. Department of Commerce, Economics and Statistics Administration: US Census Bureau.

Versényi, A. (1993), *Theatre in Latin America: Religion, Politics, and Culture from Cortés to the 1980s*, New York: Cambridge University Press.

——— (2004), 'Theatre as a Wild Weed', *Theatre Journal*, 56:3 (October), pp. 454–456.

Withey, J. A. (1971), 'Research in Asian Theatre: An Indian Model', *Educational Theatre Journal*, 23:2 (May), pp. 127–134.

Websites

Application for Employer Identification Number. http://www.ehow.com/ how_4898564_nonprofit-tax-id-number.html. Accessed 11 April 2010).

Cara Mía Theatre Company. http://caramiatheatre.com.

Dallas Office of Cultural Affairs. http://dallasculture.org.

U.S. Population Projections: 2005–2050. Pew Hispanic Center, http://pewhispanic.org/ reports/ report.php?ReportID=85, 2.11.2008. Accessed 2 May 2010).

Quick facts. http://www.quickfacts.census.gov/qfd/states/48000. Accessed 27 February 2010).

Arizona State law SB1070. http://cnmnewsnetwork.com/112197/arizona-immigration-law-sb1070-2010-and-american-protests-and-rallies/, and http://www.nytimes.com/2010/04/24/us/politics/24immig.html, for the actual Bill see http://www.azleg.gov/legtext/49leg/2r/bills/sb1070p.htm. Accessed 9 May 2010).

The Univisión Television Group. http://corporate.univision.com/corp/en/utg.jsp. Accessed 10 April 2010).

Teatro Dallas. http://www.teatrodallas.org

Notes

1 Thanks to Lisa Penaloza of EDHEC Business School, Lille, France for pointing this issue out to me and kindly sharing her own research as well as bibliographic references. Please see Penaloza's 'Immigrant Consumers: Marketing and Public Policy Considerations in the Global Economy', *Journal of Public Policy & Marketing*, 14:1 (1995), pp. 83–94; 'Atravesando Fronteras/Border Crossings: A Critical Ethnographic Exploration of the Consumer Acculturation of Mexican Immigrants', *Journal of Consumer Research* 21:1 (June 1994), pp. 32–54; with Judith Cavazos Arroyos, 'Here, There, and Beyond: Remittances in Transnational Family Consumption', *Teor'a y Praxis*, 10, pp. 131–161.

2 The Univisión Television Group owns and operates 19 full-power and seven low-power stations that provide the core distribution of the Univision Network in key markets, including Los Angeles, New York, Miami, Houston, Dallas, Chicago, San Antonio, Phoenix, San Francisco, Sacramento, Fresno, Philadelphia, Washington DC, Atlanta, Austin, Tucson, Bakersfield, Salt Lake City, Raleigh and Cleveland. The Univision Television Group stations are the No. 1 Spanish-language stations in their markets and frequently out delivers the English-language stations in total delivery of key demographics in the nation's top television markets. In addition to the Univision Television Group owned and operated stations, the Univision Network is also distributed through 64 broadcast television affiliates and 1357 cable and Direct Broadcast Satellite (DBS) affiliates nationwide.

(Quoted from their official website http://corporate.univision.com/corp/en/utg.jsp)

3 The US Census 2010 form actually states the following options: Question 8. 'Is Person 1 of Hispanic, Latino, or Spanish origin?' The response options are: 'No, not of Hispanic, Latino, or Spanish origin'; 'Yes, Mexican, Mexican Am., Chicano'; 'Yes, Puerto Rican'; 'Yes, Cuban'; 'Yes, another Hispanic, Latino, or Spanish origin – print origin, for example, Argentinean, Colombian, Dominican, Nicaraguan, Salvadoran, Spaniard, and so on.' Question 9 deals with race. 'What is Person 1's race? White; Black, African Am., or Negro; American Indian or Alaska Native – print name of principal tribe; or Asian Indian, Chinese, Japanese, Filipino, Japanese, Korean, Vietnamese, Native Hawaiian, Guamanian

or Chamorro, Samoan, Other Pacific Islander, or Some Other Race – print race.' Printed by the US Department of Commerce, Economics and Statistics Administration, US Census Bureau, 2010.

4   My collection of short stories in Spanish entitled *Entre la Argentina y Cuba: Cuentos nómadas de viajes y tangos* (*Between Argentina and Cuba: Nomad Stories of Travels and Tangos*) was published in Buenos Aires by Corregidor (2009). From a series of eight stories published here, I developed a play entitled *La familia*, which debut in Dallas in October–November 2009 at SOLART Studio and at the Bath House Cultural Center, Dallas. It was produced by the Spanish-language theatre company Cambalache Teatro en Español, a participant of this study, of which I am a member. I have also a novel in English under consideration entitled *Caribbean Blue: A Fictional Story of a Cuban Balsero.*

5   See the recent debate of Arizona State law SB1070, which many think will lead to illegal racial profiling. For public opinion regarding the law, see http://cnmnewsnetwork.com/112197/arizona-immigration-law-sb1070-2010-and-american-protests-and-rallies/; and http://www.nytimes.com/2010/04/24/us/politics/24immig.html, for the actual Bill see http://www.azleg.gov/legtext/49leg/2r/bills/sb1070p.htm.

6   The University of North Texas provides students and professors with free access to JSTOR, an electronic media resource, which made it possible for me to comb through a significant number of journal issues from the comfort of my home computer.

7   See http://quickfacts.census.gov/qfd/states/00000.html.

8   See Adam Versény's landmark *Theatre in Latin America: Religion, Politics, and Culture from Cortés to the 1980s*, New York: Cambridge University Press, 1993.

9   See publication noted above: 2.11.2008, U.S. *Population Projections: 2005–2050*, Pew Hispanic Center, http://pewhispanic.org/reports/report.php?ReportID=85. 'The Latino population, already the nation's largest minority group, will triple in size and will account for most of the nation's population growth from 2005 through 2050. Hispanics will make up 29% of the U.S. population in 2050, compared with 14% in 2005.'

10 To qualify for public funding in the United States, cultural groups must have 501(c)3 Federal Tax exempt status. In order to attain this status, organisations need to file articles of incorporation in the state of residence. This requires the employment of a lawyer, some of whom do work at reduced rates. Also, groups need to complete IRS form SS-4, 'Application for Employer Identification Number' to get a federal employer identification number (EIN). Allow up to ten weeks for the application to be processed. See, for instance, http://www.ehow.com/how_4898564_nonprofit-tax-id-number.html.

11 As part of its International Book Fair, for instance, my Spanish-language play, *La familia*, was performed in October 2010. Among others, Centro Cultural Argentino and Flor Candela have performed at the Library venue as well.

12 On May 14 2010, I served as a grant evaluator panellist for Level IV organisations (the largest dollar amount budgets) for the Dallas Office of Cultural Affairs. Organisations reviewed included Dallas Children's Theatre, Dallas Theatre Center, Dallas Opera, Dallas City Ballet, etc. For funding criteria, see www.dallas.cgweb.org, 'City of Dallas, Office of Cultural Affairs 2010–2011 CPP Guidelines'. I wanted to witness the process from the inside. Since there were no Hispanic organisations under consideration in my group, there was no conflict of

interest. Judgments by panellists were to follow 'Program Goals' (see website). The process is rather lengthy. Panellists were given web access to the grants solicitors prior to the meeting. Soliciting organisations prepared detailed budget and activities reports; seven panellists plus city officials met at the Latino Cultural Center where each soliciting organisation made an oral/visual presentation of 15 minutes, including Q&A. Panellists then rated each organisation in secret ballot. We were instructed to follow 'Program Goals', and not to be persuaded by other factors, such as perceived economic need. Each organisation was judged individually and not against each other. The Panel ratings were tallied immediately after each presentation on a computer program. At the end of the seven-hour process, organisations were projected on screen by ranking. Panellists had an opportunity to discuss the results and modify their scores, if they wished. Most of us did not. The results are subsequently handed to the Dallas Mayor's Office, whereby the Dallas City Council decides the actual dollar amount to be awarded to each organisation.

13 *Crystal City, 1969* was based on the testimonial of Diana Serna Aguilera, José Angel Gutiérrez (now Professor of Political Science at the University of Texas, Arlington), Serevita Lara (present librarian at Crystal City High School) and Mario Treviño.

14 *Cambalache* (from the *lunfardo*, an argot developed in the late nineteenth century in the immigrant-laden port of Buenos Aires) is a polyphonic term that means: an exchange of second-hand goods at a street fair, an exchange made with the objective of getting the upper hand, and it is also a tango composed in 1943 by Argentinean poet Enrique Santos Discépolo, describing the changing times at the turn of the last century.

Chapter 9

Challenging Racial Categorisation Through Theatre: English-language Theatre in Malaysia

Susan Philip

While today 'race' is a generally discredited term, in Malaysia it continues to be socially relevant, because of the way in which Malaysian society has been constructed as well as the ways in which race has been defined and used within the Malaysian context. Race was established as a central marker of identity in colonial times, and is still treated as such for everyday transactions. However, more and more, individuals are beginning to take issue with the ways in which race is defined by the authorities, and even with the need to categorise people by race at all. This has led to increasing contestation of and negotiation with these authority-defined categories. As Les Back and John Solomos point out, '[…] "races" are created within the context of political and social regulation. Thus "race" is above all a political construct' (Back and Solomos 2000: 8). It can, therefore, be constructed in ways which oppose, or at the very least question, the dominant constructions. The English-language theatre of Malaysia has long been a site within which challenges to dominant discourse have been embodied and played out; in this chapter, I will focus specifically on how this theatre has dealt with issues of race and racial identity since Independence.

Living in Malaysia, one cannot escape the issue of race. Every Malaysian is required to 'have' a race; there is an official list of four races to choose from, namely Malay, Chinese, Indian and Other. While 'Malay', 'Chinese' and 'Indian' are all defined by language use, culture and religion, 'Chinese' and 'Indian' are further determined by paternal ancestry traced back to China or India; 'Other' refers to all who cannot be accommodated in the other three categories. This narrow racial label is required for many day-to-day transactions (such as opening a bank account), and is embedded in the identity card which all citizens from the age of twelve must carry.[1] Increasingly, racial and cultural hybridity are being acknowledged within society as a reality; but this hybridity constantly comes up against the brick wall of authoritative discourse which functions by the vocabulary of separation and difference, self and other. What I will look at in this chapter is how negotiations with these complex and conflicting ideas take place through the theatre – specifically the English-language theatre which has, from its earliest days, dealt with issues of race, identity and belonging.

Race in Malaysia

In the Malaysian context, the superior/inferior binary which informed the racial rhetoric of the colonisers has been replaced by the rhetoric of belonging/non-belonging. In Malaysia, belonging to a specific racial group is central to having greater access to power and ownership;

the Malays, defined as native to Malaysia, are seen as the 'owners' of the land. With this ownership comes greater political power as well as certain economic and social privileges. It is therefore important for the state to be able to unambiguously define who is and who is not a Malay. There is no room in this framework for the ambiguity of hybrid racial identities, which upset the fictive neatness of the boundaries drawn by the authorities. However, rigid racial categorisation is actually a fairly recent phenomenon in Malaysia's history, beginning in the nineteenth century.

In order to reap the wealth of Malaya, the British administration in the nineteenth century imported labour from India and China. The Malays, whom the British regarded as native to Malaya, were left to work their own land or, if they were aristocrats, began to be educated in English with a view to turning out suitable civil servants. Amarjit Kaur points out that 'the colonial authorities deliberately chose to adopt the segmentation of labour along racial lines. This allowed them to play off one racial group against another' (Kaur 2001: 189). Thus, communalism and distrust of, and distance from, 'other' races meant that racial hybridity came to be regarded with suspicion both by the colonisers and later, by the postcolonial government; it gradually became less acceptable, and the idea of belonging to just one particular race took root among the early migrants to Malaya.

The notion of race began to be narrowed down and concretised through the work of census takers. Both Nirmala PuruShotam and Charles Hirschman have written on this phenomenon. PuruShotam writes in the context of British Singapore, but her comments are relevant for British Malaya as well. She sees the whole census-taking process as 'naming and related meaning-making practices' (PuruShotam 1998: 57) engineered by the dominant group.

This legacy of British census-taking activities left the post-Independence government with a handy tool for categorising the peoples of Malaysia, thus 'naming' them and 'making meaning' about them according to the political and national needs of the time. For example, post-independence citizenship was extended to all by right of birth on Malayan soil, even for those of immigrant ancestry. However, 'final acceptance of this provision [by the Malay leaders] was only obtained in return for a guarantee of Malay privileges' (Andaya and Andaya 2001: 276). This indicates a perceived need among the Malays to protect themselves and their territory from outside encroachment; which also implies the need to define 'self' and 'other' as well as 'insider' and 'outsider'. In this context, it is pertinent to note Hirschman's assertion that 'the residue of racial ideology continues to haunt contemporary Malaysia' (Hirschman 1987: 570); even though overtly racist thinking in terms of the 'superior/inferior' binary was not part of the hammering out of the terms of independence, there is clearly still some sense of fear of 'others' inherent within this racialised social framework. This fear is strongest in the authorities, who depend on the fixity of racial categorisation as a means of maintaining their power base. Hybridity is to be avoided as hybrid identities transgress all manner of racial, cultural and linguistic barriers, thus bringing into question the validity of the constructed boundaries.

There is opposition to these rigid notions of racial identity. Farish Noor, a prominent scholar and commentator on Malaysia, suggests moving '[t]owards an abstract Malaysian citizenship' (Noor 2008: 17), rather than one predicated on race. A Malay rubber smallholder declares that his family 'have traditionally been PAS[2] supporters. I voted PAS because Umno is a Malay party, PAS an Islamic party. Umno is communal-based; PAS dispenses justice to all regardless of race' (Kee 2008: 319). At many levels of society, then, the willingness to be bound by the requirements of narrow definitions of race and communalism is slowly loosening and being challenged in interesting ways. Playwright Huzir Sulaiman, for example, chose to re-define himself racially, changing his official race from 'Malay' to 'Indian', underlining the constructedness of categories which, in Malaysia, are treated as inherent.[3] Officially categorised as Malay, Huzir questions the factual and logical validity of the classification, and demonstrates its ungroundedness by deliberately choosing a more 'appropriate' race. And yet he still questions the validity of what he has himself chosen. Ultimately, he says, there is nothing in his life other than historical precedent to anchor him to the choice he has made. And, pertinently, echoing Farish Noor's statement, he asks if there is a need to make such a choice, to label oneself. Is the wider and more inclusive label of nationality not enough? A kind of Malaysianness that questions and sometimes even transcends race is portrayed and debated in the theatre, suggesting a strong resistance to authoritative impositions of racial identity.

Post-independence theatre: The 1960s and the search for a national identity

Because ownership of and belonging to the nation have been stated in such clear-cut, racialised terms (Malays belong to and own the land, others do not), it became clear that political and economic power were also being perceived in racialised terms. A sampling of drama from the late 1960s and early 1970s, particularly the plays anthologised in *New Drama One*, shows that racial identities and racial tensions were of central concern to many Malaysians. Edward Dorall's *A Tiger is Loose in Our Community* (1967), for example, depicts a multiracial community, showing the underlying racially fuelled tensions which beset his characters, who live in a squatter village.

Dorall's depiction of the squatter area seems to suggest at first a kind of unity. All the inhabitants are united by the drabness and poverty of their surroundings. They are shown whiling away their time, arranged in small multiracial groupings. However, hostilities break out quickly and easily among these apparently harmonious groups. An interesting point is that as soon as racial tensions start to surface, the characters quickly retreat into their own vernaculars, insulting each other in Malay, Tamil and Cantonese. Mutual incomprehensibility serves to cut them off from each other, and takes away any possibility of establishing communication. This seems to echo Ghulam-Sarwar Yousof's point that Malaysians cannot move beyond 'the cultural and particularly linguistic "shells" within which they live [...] because they do not understand any culture but their own' (Yousof 1982: 22). Lacking common ground, they retreat into their authority-defined racial and linguistic boxes, shouting at each other in languages essentially foreign to each other.

The propensity towards communalism easily tips over into racism. Any attempt to overcome these racist responses is defeated by pervasive hostility. One character, Kali, has a transcendent vision of what their society could be – lush orchards where goats and tigers declare their love for each other. But in the end, rather than allowing this vision to flourish, the vengeful inhabitants of the squatter area manipulate events so that Kali and the local gangster fight, with both of them ending up dead.

Lee Joo For's *The Happening in the Bungalow* (1970) also presents a potentially utopian vision, undercut again by hatred and calls for violence and blood. It focuses on events occurring 'somewhere in West Malaysia during an early month of 1969',[4] particularly on the relationships and manoeuverings among Rozni (a Malay woman), Cheng (a Chinese man) and Birch (an Englishman, now a Malaysian citizen). The name 'Birch' would be significant to a Malaysian audience, being the surname of J. W. W. Birch, the first British Resident of Perak; Birch, who caused unhappiness among Perak's Malay chiefs with his manner of handling matters they regarded as their traditional right, was assassinated by these chiefs. The incident has been viewed as an early manifestation of Malay nationalism (Andaya and Andaya 2001: 166). This, juxtaposed with the oblique reference to May 1969, suggests that the author is attempting to interrogate nationalism and belonging in Malaysia.

Lee puts forward two visions of nationalism in this play. First, there is the naively inclusive and welcoming vision of Rozni. This is contrasted with the violence and hatred of a mob that has gathered outside, and ultimately the picture of the mob dominates. Birch steps out to confront them and is killed. Their presence is palpable throughout the rest of the play. While Rozni declares an open welcome for all, this mob (not specified by race) is outside the bungalow, chanting threats such as 'Kill – kill – kill the other kind of people!' and 'Fight back! Kill the others! Blood for blood! Kill! Kill! Kill!' (Lee 1972: 143). Rozni's belief that everyone shares equally in the nation is severely undermined by the demands for blood of the 'others'. It is interesting that we cannot apportion blame by race – implying that Lee is indicting all who continue to hold on to this racialised view which insists on the self/other binary.

In both plays, the writers display a fundamental uncertainty about the place of 'others' within the Malaysian nation. They demonstrate the frailty and vulnerability of individuals (like Kali, Rozni and Cheng) who seek to step beyond their specified borders to reach towards a more inclusive vision; their voices are drowned out by the voices calling for division and separation, and for violence towards the other. This reflected the lack of certainty which characterised the immediate post-independence period, when the guidelines for citizenship had just been formulated and were still being 'tested'. Belonging within the nation was still being negotiated, but was destabilised by the threat of racial violence. By the 1980s, the question of belonging had not been fully resolved, though there was a determination on the part of some to work towards a form of cultural expression which did not function by divisive racial categories – that is, to take ownership of their cultural identities by working beyond mere racial categories.

The 1980s: Finding common cultural ground?

The 1970s, with the implementation of the National Language Policy and the concretising of the National Cultural Policy, saw a slowdown in English-language writing in Malaysia. The National Language Policy set Malay as the national language and, later, as the main language for education. The National Cultural Policy, meanwhile, declared that:

i. Malaysia's national culture must be based on the indigenous culture of the people of this region.
ii. Elements of other cultures which are suitable and appropriate can be incorporated into the national culture.
iii. Islam is an important element in the formation of the national culture.

(Affandi Hassan 1973: vii)[5]

Many non-Malay writers chose to leave Malaysia, feeling that these new policies implied that there was no place for them in the nation as it was then being articulated. What place was there, they wondered, for non-Malays in a society which so determinedly foregrounded the Malay language and Malay culture? What sense of belonging could there be, for those of another race? Not only were these questions actively debated through the theatre during the 1980s, but the theatre also began to work towards trying to create that sense of belonging, as well as of ownership of a common culture.

In the 1980s, some concerned individuals formed groups which began to consciously work toward a more Malaysian aesthetic in the theatre. Chief among these groups was the Five Arts Centre (FAC), an arts collective founded in 1984 which aimed 'to give the performing arts a Malaysian identity' (Arfah 2004). One of the founding members, influential director and critic Krishen Jit, states that he 'wanted to show a sense of what it was like living here, what is happening here. A sense of difference between what is official, what is public, what is private, what is alternative' (Jhybe 2001). The desire to examine the liminal spaces between official and alternative meant not only dealing with works which focused on issues of race and culture, but also finding new performance modes. The FAC is known for producing works which experiment with movement, music and ideas, with the specific aim of 'articulating multiple Malaysian identities' (Five Arts Centre). The focus on multiple identities challenges the authoritative pronouncement that each racialised individual must claim a specific essentialised cultural identity. The narrowness of the official outlook on race and culture is made clear in a comment made about dancer Marion D'Cruz (one of the founder members of FAC, and racially categorised as 'Indian'), who actively engaged with Malay dance forms: she remembers that 'one famous comment came out in a magazine that said, "Budak India tidak boleh menari Melayu", which basically means, "An Indian child cannot dance Malay"' (quoted in Brownell 2009). This is an attitude which seeks to bar 'others' from entering into that which has been defined as 'Malay' space, thus valorising 'purity' over hybridity. FAC, however, chose to step beyond the boundaries of purity in order to seek a common cultural space.

However, this desire to maintain purity remains dominant in society, and is reflected and challenged in two seminal works from the 1980s, Kee Thuan Chye's *1984 Here and Now* and K. S. Maniam's *The Cord*. Both writers believe strongly in the need for Malaysians to embrace the multiple cultures surrounding them, as a step towards articulating a more holistic rather than narrowly race-based Malaysian identity. Maniam opposes rigid labelling according to race, arguing instead for the development of a 'common mental and imaginative space' (Maniam 2001: 10). Kee, similarly, complains of people 'who do not want to embrace pluralism, multiculturalism – the idea of Bangsa Malaysia'[6] (Kee 2006: 4).

Both *1984 Here and Now* and *The Cord* examine deeply segregated societies. Kee's play is openly politically engaged, using allegory to examine race-based political and social ideologies and policies. Maniam's work appears to be more communal, focusing as it does on a part of the Indian community; but his examination of the lives of Indian plantation workers engages with the consequences of the implementation of race-based political ideologies.

Kee's play, as is obvious from the title, references George Orwell's *1984*. It was staged in 1985 at the University of Malaya's Experimental Theatre, and ran for five nights (at a time when two or three nights was the norm). On the last three nights, performances were completely sold out, word having got round that this play dealt in a barely veiled way with issues of race, privilege and marginalisation usually deemed too sensitive to talk about. Reviewer Kit Lee saw the play as 'at least one fine crack in the monolith of authoritarianism' (Kit Lee 1987: v), a challenge to the 'unquestionable' business of linking race and privilege. Kee himself saw the play as questioning the marginalisation of races which had played a part in the development of the nation: 'Our forefathers made this land prosper – they AND we should not be forgotten. I long for the sense of belonging and the spirit of resilience that come with a genuine respect for the human being' (Kee 1987: ii).

Although this play has an overtly political agenda, race is central to the discussion because of how party politics are structured in Malaysia. The government has, since Independence, been made up of a coalition of predominantly race-based political parties.[7] Within this coalition, UMNO is the dominant partner; in any general election, it is understood that if the BN wins, the president of UMNO will be Prime Minister. Thus in Malaysia, political power is specifically tied to race. Because of this it is possible to read Kee's play, which centres around struggles between the Malays/Party members (who are privileged within this social framework) and the Chinese/Proles (who are marginalised), as also being about race and power.

There are no specific references within the play which situate it in Malaysia, or indeed any other recognisable country. However, the rhetoric used clearly points to the situation within Malaysia. In the first scene, for example, the Big Brother character declares:

The Party is supreme. It will strive for the rights of the Party members, for their place of ascendancy in the nation. Party members must unite, one and all with no exception. As for the Proles who have made their homes in this nation, we welcome them to stay. But they must understand that, above all else, the Party members must be kept happy The Party members must not feel threatened or deprived in this land that is rightfully theirs.

(Kee 1987: 3)

This is all too reminiscent of rhetoric that has appeared time and again in the Malaysian newspapers, reminding the non-Malays of their origins elsewhere. This, coupled with the idea that the Party members (who view the nation as 'theirs') are the centre, and the Proles the immigrant 'other', makes it clear to a Malaysian audience that the action of the play actually speaks about the situation in Malaysia. And because the political situation in Malaysia is so tied to notions of race, the play turns into a debate about race and belonging within the nation. However, rather than just turning this discussion into a complaint against the dominant race, Kee targets narrow communal thinking at all levels.

Kee's play includes characters who seek to rise above communal thinking. For instance the hero, Wiran,[8] falls in love with Yone, a Prole woman (it is implied that Wiran is of the right race to be a Party member). They are kept apart by the prejudices of both Party members and Proles. Wiran, for example, is arrested and accused of disgracing his own race (Kee 1987: 76); when Yone comes home late, saying she was at a party with a friend, her father snarlingly demands to know 'Wat race? ... Hnarh? ... Wat race?' (Kee 1987: 43).

Sadly, the impression left at the end of the play is of persecution, fear and uncertainty, overcoming any hope of a relationship between Wiran and Yone. In the last scene, Wiran bursts into the auditorium, apparently on the run from his jailers. He addresses the audience, trying to incite them to action:

WIRAN: Are you all going to sit here and do nothing? The hope of this nation lies with you! Are you going to sit here and let it go to the dogs? Stand up! Stand up and unite! Party members, Proles, whoever you are, wherever you are. Speak up for your rights! This is a democracy. Stand up for your freedom, for racial equality and integration, for humanity and justice, for truth, for a nation capable of greatness!

(Kee 1987: 88)

It is then left up to the audience to decide whether or not they will save him from the police. The last thing the audience sees before the blackout is the police, relentlessly pursuing Wiran. They are left, then, with the impression of the anti-racist hero on the verge of being punished for his stance.

Kee's presentation of racism and communalism in this society fall back into stereotypes, reflective of the very broad and essentialised ways in which Malaysians often think about race themselves. However, director Krishen Jit subverted ideas of racial essentialism through his decision to cast across racial barriers. Thus Big Brother and high-ranking Party member Shadrin were played by Indian actors; Yone was played by an actor of mixed Malay and Chinese parentage who, because of the way racial definition works in Malaysia, is considered Malay. Lo points out the 'deconstructive potential of such a performance' (Lo 2004: 88):

race, considered such an immutable category, is shown through the racially transgressive casting to be a fluid and mutable.

K. S. Maniam's play portrays one racial community but, oddly, reaches beyond ideas of communalism more effectively than does Kee's play. Staged in 1984, the play centres around a group of workers in a rubber plantation, focusing particularly on the tensions between Muniandy, his son Ratnam, and the supervisor Muthiah. Historically, labourers on plantations in Malaysia have been Indian (Tamils). First brought over from India by the British as indentured labourers, many of them stayed and had families; subsequent generations then continued to work on the plantations. There was little need to leave the plantations, as food, schools and medical services were all available (though their quality can be disputed). Indians (mainly Malayalis and those of Sri Lankan extraction) were also prominent as plantation administrators. Here, inter-ethnic tensions, often carried over from India, tended to dominate; thus despite the potential for unity implied by the broad racial category 'Indian', there was in fact a great deal of distrust and division among the labourers and the administrators. This reality in itself undermines the validity and relevance of authority-defined racial categories.

It is a reality Maniam deals with in his play. Muthiah, the young administrator, persecutes manual labourer Muniandy, the first-generation migrant. Initially respectful towards Muniandy, Muthiah quickly allows his greater access to power to dominate and distort their relationship. He betrays Muniandy by raping his wife – Ratnam is actually the product of that rape, though Muniandy is initially unaware of this. By confronting these issues of betrayal and power, Maniam refuses easy notions of intra-ethnic/racial unity. Instead, through Ratnam and Muniandy, he suggests that it is necessary to step beyond racial borders towards a more hybrid and inclusive identity. Ratnam needs to take his place as a member of what Maniam calls the 'new diaspora':

Unlike the traditional diaspora, the new diaspora consists of men and women dispersed among various cultural communities, and who seek another, more liberated cultural community. Exiled within their own homelands, they construct and live within a common mental and imaginative space. This common mental and imaginative space is not arbitrarily or mechanically put together; it evolves from the recognition that man has been artificially categorised into a monocultural, ethnic and political being when multiplicity is his true nature.

(Maniam 2001: 10)

The closed, almost monocultural world of the plantation can be read as representing Malaysian society as constructed by the authorities; it symbolises the authoritative demand that each individual be, as Maniam says, 'artificially categorised into a monocultural [...] being'; Ratnam, born and brought up within the confines of the plantation, now longs 'to go from this place. There must be a future somewhere else' (Maniam 1994: 89). Muthiah, aware that Ratnam is his son, has tried to teach him English, the language of authority on the plantation, but according to Muniandy, 'something rebelled in him. He hated your authority' (Maniam 1994: 92). If we see Muthiah as representative of the authorities within the plantation, then he also reflects the authorities within Malaysia who seek to categorise according to narrow labels. Ratnam rejects this authority, just as he rejects the language of power which Muthiah tries to give him. Instead, when he uses English, he speaks in what Maniam calls 'pidgin English', and what Ratnam calls 'real-life English':

> RATNAM: Now the language is spoke like I can speak it. *(He goes into pidgin English.)* 'You want go jamban' not 'Could you show me the bathroom, please!' You can talk to me in the language we all know. I can speak real-life English now.
>
> (Maniam 1994: 64)

Ratnam's rejection of Muthiah's language (standard English) and his authority, as well as his desire to escape from the confines of the plantation, indicate a desire to go beyond the closed, monocultural world he currently inhabits. This implies a desire to transcend mere racial boundaries to find a space within Malaysian society that can accommodate the fact of his hybridity. This reflects the desire of individuals within the nation to also discard limited and limiting categories such as race. Kee, by highlighting the ugliness of racial chauvinism, and Maniam, by demonstrating its limitations and pointing to a more hybrid racial and cultural identity, both emphasise the urgency of finding common ground that stands outside the borders of racial identification. However, as my examination of the plays *Stories for Amah* and *Gold Rain and Hailstones* (both written in the 1990s) will indicate, this desire has clearly not come to fruition.

The 1990s: Venturing beyond labels

Where writers in the 1960s and 1970s, and to some extent the 1980s, were questioning the relevance of race within the larger context of national identity, writers in the 1990s have looked at race in a much narrower and more specific way. It is important to note that neither playwright in this section questions his belonging within the nation. Now, the aim seems to be to loosen the bonds of the straitjacket that is racial identification in Malaysia. The two writers examined in this section interrogate the actual meaning of the race labels they have been given, confronting the monolithic definition with their own fluid hybridity. Malay writer Jit Murad deals with a group – privileged, overseas-educated Malays – whom he considers to be marginalised within the Malaysian social framework because they do not adhere to an essentialised definition of Malayness, while Eurasian writer Mark de Silva questions whether paternal descent is enough to racially and culturally categorise a person.

Malaysians do not often question the racial category 'Malay', because it falls under the rubric of potentially 'sensitive' topics. It is the only racial category to be defined in the constitution, according to which a Malay is someone who speaks the Malay language, habitually practices Malay customs, and professes Islam as his or her religion (Article 160, Malaysian constitution). The category, while 'defined', is oddly open and inclusive – according to this definition, anyone who follows the above guidelines can be considered Malay, regardless of paternal or maternal lineage. Although belonging to any of the other racial categories is dependent on paternal descent, the 'Malay' category is more concerned about religious affiliation. Thus if a Malay-Muslim woman has a child with a Chinese man, the child will be categorised as Malay and Muslim, not according to paternal descent. Clearly, the boundaries of Malayness are fluid and shifting, although treated as monolithic and fixed. However, Malayness is increasingly coming to be seen as a monolithic identity, therefore also becoming less open and inclusive.

In *Gold Rain and Hailstones*, playwright Jit Murad examines the marginalisation of Malays who, through class and education, are openly hybrid in terms of culture and language use. Specifically, he looks at privileged middle- to upper-middle-class Malays who have been educated abroad, and who return to Malaysia to find that they must negotiate a space for their hybrid selves within the essentialised category 'Malay'.

The problem that these young people face is that they do not necessarily follow Malay customs, nor do they speak the Malay language. But as one character notes, there are 'a lot more of us than you'd think. We Melayu "Speaking", "Celup"' (Murad: 1). The word 'speaking' as Jit uses it here implies that they are Malays who speak 'differently' – not only using English, but probably with unusual fluency, or marked by a non-Malaysian accent. But this group not only uses English, it mixes it with Malay to create a fluent, energetic bilingualism which could only have been born in Malaysia. 'Celup' is a Malay word referring to the process of plating jewellery in gold, and implies that a person has a false veneer of foreignness. Both terms are derogatory in tone. There is a sense, then, that the use of English is a kind of false coat, a layer that hides the essential, 'real' Malay.

But does linguistic and cultural hybridity mean that they can no longer claim racial belonging? Are they any less Malay than those who are more compliant? The issue is primarily debated through the characters Jay and Amy. Amy is a prickly, confrontational perpetual graduate student who has remained in America. On returning home, she immediately finds herself out of place because she doesn't dress modestly and doesn't speak Malay. Jay wrestles with the problem of being gay in a society which does not recognise homosexuality and criminalises 'sodomy'. Thus both of them are outside the borders of the official definition of Malayness.

Amy's response is to get upset by the way in which mainstream Malays respond to her. She is angered that people stare at her when she wears a somewhat revealing halter top, and discovers to her cost that if 'you enter a government office, and you're Malay but don't speak it, it had better be because you're mute' (Murad: 17). Because of the rigidity of the definition on matters of language and religion, people like Amy who have taken on elements of other cultures find themselves excluded from their own racial category.

Jay's response is more practical. Aware that he must just survive and get along in this very narrow society, he adopts whatever cultural elements he needs, when he needs them. Thus, he speaks excellent colloquial Malay, and his sexual identity must remain closeted and unacknowledged in public. Yet, as a television host for a programme on beauty and makeup, he hints subtextually at his homosexuality. Jay fragments himself, projecting one identity in public, another among friends, and yet another when he is on holiday abroad.

The Malaysian social framework, with its insistence on unproblematic categories of race, refuses both these characters the space in which to express and embody their hybridity; there is an 'essential' Malayness to which they are expected to conform. Amy finally rejects this idea, realising that 'the more you define yourself, the less space you have to live' (Murad: 66). The authoritative urge to define has certainly narrowed the spaces where Amy and Jay can comfortably live. Amy decides that she must continue to be her hybrid self, uncomfortable as it is, to make people aware 'that different things are born here and grow here, and eventually, room must be made' (Murad: 66).

Interestingly, as an examination of Mark de Silva's *Stories for Amah* will show, the authoritative drive to essentialise can be internalised even within a racial category which is by definition hybrid. In *Stories for Amah*, we get a complex and layered examination of the ways in which categorisation works, and how individuals can be complicit in limiting and racialising their own identities, even within the boundaries set by the state. De Silva, who is officially labelled as Eurasian, brings to light how difficult and, more importantly, damaging it can be to insist on confining individuals within large, essentialised definitions of race.

As mentioned earlier, the Eurasians are ethnically hybrid; most people in Malaysia who are labelled 'Eurasian' have a history in the region dating back four or five hundred years, with the first Portuguese settlers in the region. These original Portuguese settlers often married locally, and the result today is this ethnically very complex group which defies labelling by the normal procedures. Even within the Eurasian community, there is questioning and argument over who can be considered a 'true' Eurasian – with, for example, some Portuguese Eurasians unwilling to consider those of Dutch or English ancestry as Eurasians. The national habit of defining borders has become so deeply ingrained that even groups which are undeniably hybrid, seem to seek after essentialising classifications.

Stories for Amah, written and first staged in 2002 by the Actors Studio in Kuala Lumpur, deals with an Eurasian girl, Ruth de Souza, who must learn to negotiate between the Chinese culture of her mother and grandmother, in which she has been brought up, and the Eurasian culture of her father, which is later imposed on her. The playwright presents her father and his insistence on the patriarchal culture as overbearing, imposing an essentially alien culture on Ruth by demanding that she 'be' Eurasian. Because her father is Eurasian, that must also be her official racial category. But this label clearly ignores the Chinese influence on her in terms of language and culture. Thus, although her official label is actually hybrid, the practice of categorisation at the official level works to narrowly define her actual hybridity. Able to claim both her Eurasian and Chinese heritages, Ruth is constrained to choose only one label. 'Eurasians' are treated as a monolithic and homogeneous group despite the vast differences that can clearly exist within individuals. Having been affixed with that label, Ruth is not allowed to 'be' Chinese, even though her upbringing has in fact left her feeling culturally and linguistically Chinese.

Of particular interest in this play is the way in which the Eurasian characters seek to define their almost impenetrably hybrid racial identities so that they seem less hybrid. For example, Uncle Zack perceives himself to be in a different (superior) racial category from Ruth's father despite the fact that they are cousins, purely because Ruth's mother is Chinese, while Uncle Zack's wife is 'half Dutch, so she is a real Eurasian' (De Silva 2002: 20). The implication seems to be that by adding this extra, non-Eurasian element of hybridity, the 'purity' of the Eurasian heritage has been diluted.

De Silva's play in many ways accurately reflects the complexities of racial categorisation in Malaysia – the pre-conceptions about different races, the urge to essentialise, the hostility towards 'others', the perceived need to maintain racial boundaries and, underlying it all, the sheer arbitrariness of many of these labels and narrowly bordered spaces. At the end of the play he has Ruth declare that: 'my voice is slowly coming, and I can slowly tok and fight back alredi [...] that voice don have a colour, and don have a name, is just a voice that you help me find, and a voice that you now put in me [...]' (De Silva 2002: 59). This declaration, with its emphasis on transcending race labels, is also reminiscent of Jit's assertion that room must be made for racially and culturally transgressive 'mutants'.

Conclusion

In terms of size, population and economy, Malaysia is unquestionably a small nation. However, I would argue that it is also a small nation in terms of how it deals with issues of race. Situated in a geographical location which has led to its constantly being exposed to a myriad cultural and racial influences, it yet seeks to retreat within narrow and limiting racial and cultural boundaries, thus imposing a kind of involuntary smallness and narrowness on its inhabitants. It turns inwards, protecting itself from the threatening hybridity of a globalised world. Economically open to trade from the rest of the world, Malaysia nonetheless seems to want to refuse to allow the attendant exchange of culture and development of hybrid cultures to occur. Its putative cultural purities must be maintained.

In the final analysis, it becomes clear that race and racial labelling are still a deeply entrenched part of Malaysian life. Despite a clear change in attitudes, as shown by this chronological examination of how the issue of race is dealt with in the English-language theatres of Malaysia, the fact remains that race as a construct has taken deep root in the Malaysian psyche. The concept has been internalised by the majority of the population; constant repetition at the authoritative level helps to cement that internalisation to the point where it is deemed both natural and right. The dissenting voices, such as those presented here, are a minority, and this is reflected in the overall pessimism of tone of the authors. However, the works examined here represent a vital attempt to bring issues of race into a kind of open, public debate. How long such debate will take to unsettle the Malaysian construction of race, is an open question.

Works cited

Affandi Hassan, M. (1973), *Asas Kebudayaan Kebangsaan*, Kuala Lumpur: Kementerian Kebudayaan, Belia dan Sukan.

Andaya, B. W., and Andaya, L. Y. (2001), *A History of Malaysia*, 2nd ed., Hampshire: Palgrave.

Arfah, S. (2004), '20 Years on and Still At It', *New Straits Times*, 7 February, Life and Times Entertainment 4. Article 160, Federal Constitution of Malaysia.

Back, L., and Solomos, J. (2000), 'Introduction: Theorising Race and Racism', in L. Back and J. Solomos (eds.), *Theories of Race and Racism: A Reader*, London and New York: Routledge.

Brownell, C. (2009), 'Battling the Lobotomy of Malaysia', http://www.thenutgraph.com/battlingthe-lobotomy-of-malaysia. Accessed 15 March 2010.

De Silva, M. (2002), *Stories for Amah. True Accounts of a 'Lain-lain' Girl*, Kuala Lumpur, Malaysia: The Actors Studio.

Dorall, E. (1972), 'A Tiger is Loose in Our Community', in Lloyd Fernando (ed.), *New Drama One*, Kuala Lumpur: Oxford University Press.

Five Arts Centre, 'Our Profile', http://www.fiveartscentre.org/about.php. Last accessed 15 March 2010.

Hirschman, C. (1987), 'The Meaning and Measurement of Ethnicity in Malaysia: An Analysis of Census Classifications', *Journal of Asian Studies*, 46:3 (August), pp. 555–582.

Huzir, S. (2009), '25 Things About Malaysia and Me', *The Star Online*, http://thestar.com.my/lifestyle/story.asp?file=/2009/2/8/lifefocus/3215187&sec=lifefocus. Accessed 2 October 2009.

Jhybe (2001), 'The Art of Being Krishen', *New Straits Times*, 22 August, Life and Times Literary 2.

Kaur, A. (2001), 'Sojourners and Settlers: South Indians and Communal Identity in Malaysia', in Crispin Bates (ed.), *Community, Empire and Migration: South Asians in Diaspora*, Hampshire: Palgrave, pp. 185–205.

Kee, T. C. (1987), 'Call a Spade a Spade', in Kee Thuan Chye (ed.), 1984, *Here and Now*, Selangor, Malaysia: K. Das. Ink, pp. i–ii.

——— (2006), 'Free to Speak. Freedom of Expression and Culture in Malaysia: Telling You What You Already Know', http://www.kakiseni.com/print/articles/features/MDk2OA.html. Accessed 30 October 2006.

——— (2008), *March 8: The Day Malaysia Woke Up*, Selangor, Malaysia: Marshall Cavendish.

Kit, L. (1987), 'Big Brother Lives: Introduction', in Kee Thuan Chye (ed.), *1984, Here and Now*, Selangor, Malaysia: K. Das Ink, pp. iii–xxi.

Lee, J. F. (1972), *The Happening in the Bungalow*, in Lloyd Fernando (ed.), *New Drama One*, Kuala Lumpur: Oxford University Press.

Lo, J. (2004), *Staging Nation: Postcolonial English Language Theatre in Malaysia and Singapore*, Hong Kong: Hong Kong University Press.

Maniam, K. S. (1994), *The Cord*, in K. S. Maniam (ed.), *Sensuous Horizons: The Stories and the Plays*, London: Skoob Books.

——— (2001), 'The New Diaspora', University of Calgary, 11 pp., 10 May, http://www.ucalgary.ca/UofC.eduweb.engl392/492a/articles.maniam-dias.html. Accessed 10 May 2001.

Murad, J. *Gold Rain and Hailstones*, Unpublished manuscript.

Noor, F. (2008), 'In Search of a Malaysian Identity, Still,' in Fong Chin Wei and Yin Ee Kiong (eds.), *Out of the Tempurung: Critical Essays on Malaysian Society*, New South Wales, Australia: East West Publishing.

PuruShotam, N. (1998), 'Disciplining Difference: Race in Singapore', in Joel S. Kahn (ed.), *Southeast Asian Identities: Culture and the Politics of Representation in Indonesia, Malaysia, Singapore and Thailand*, Singapore: Institute of Southeast Asian Studies, pp. 51–94.

Yousouf, G. S. (1982), 'Malaysian-Singapore Drama in English: Themes and Styles,' in B. Bennett, E. T. Hong and R. Shepherds (eds.), *The Writer's Sense of the Contemporary: Papers in Southeast Asian and Australian Literature*, Perth: Centre for Studies in Australian Literature, pp. 21–25.

Notes

1 The identity card was introduced as a security measure during the time of the Communist insurgency, when Emergency was declared in 1947, and has never been discarded. It details the name, address, date of birth, race and citizenship of the individual. In the latest version of the card, the individual's race does not appear; however, this information is embedded in the bar code, meaning that it can be accessed by any government agency linked to the National Registration Department's database.

2 PAS (Parti Islam Se-Malaysia) is an Islamic-based political party which is now part of the opposition alliance.

3 Huzir's article reads: 'Let me start at the beginning. My birth certificate declares my race to be Malay. However, as far as I can ascertain, out of my 16 great-great-grandparents, 15 were born in India. They were from all over: Kerala, Tamil Nadu, Maharashtra and Uttar Pradesh. The other great-great-grandparent – my mother's mother's mother's father – was a Chinese Muslim from Yarkand, an old Silk Road town in what is now Xinjiang Province. How all that makes me Malay I don't know. […] Anyway, when I started working in Singapore, I had to go and get my Identity Card there. I had to fill in a form. Under 'Citizenship' – Malaysian of course – there was a slot for "Race". Suddenly I realised that I could choose what I wanted to be. I could tick any box I liked. In 2003, at the age of 30, and in another country, I became Indian. For the next few years, as I travelled back and forth between KL and Singapore, my race would change at the border. I was Malay in Malaysia, and Indian in Singapore. Finally, when I updated my Malaysian IC to the MyKad […] I put down Indian as my "Bangsa". So now I am Indian everywhere. Or am I? I ask myself: how am I Indian? How can I justify calling myself Indian? Am I Indian just because 15 of my 16 great-great grandparents were born in India? I've only been there once. I speak no Indian language. I love Indian food – but I love Malay food equally. What Indian customs do I practise? Does spending hours in a bookshop count? Having a heavy lunch and then a nap? Arguing just for the sheer pleasure of it? Is that why I am Indian? If that's the basis for it, I might as well be Malay. Or Chinese. Or – here's a thought – just Malaysian.'

4   On 13 May 1969, bloody and deadly racial riots broke out in Malaysia. The cause of these riots has always been said to be racial tension. 'May 13' has become a byword in Malaysia for uncontrollable violence.

5   The translation is mine. The original text is as follows:

   i. Kebudayaan Kebangsaan Malaysia haruslah berasaskan kebudayaan asli rakyat rantau ini.

   ii. Unsur-unsur kebudayaan lain yang sesuai dan wajar boleh diterima menjadi unsur kebudayaan kebangsaan.

   iii. Islam menjadi unsur yang penting dalam pembentukan kebudayaan kebangsaan itu.

6   *Bangsa Malaysia* can be defined both as 'Malaysian people' and 'Malaysian race'; either way, it points to an inclusive rather than an exclusive outlook.

7   This alliance, called the *Barisan Nasional* or National Front, is made up of various mainly communally based political parties such as the MCA (Malaysian Chinese Association) and MIC (Malaysian Indian Congress). The alliance is dominated by UMNO (United Malays National Organisation).

8   'Wiran' sounds similar to 'Wira', the Malay word for 'hero'.

Chapter 10

From Springtime Erotics to Micro-nationalism: Altering Landscapes and Sentiments of the Assamese *Bihu* dance in North-east India

Aparna Sharma

So dear is the muga[1] bobbin,
So dear the shuttle,
Dearer still is Bohag Bihu,
How can we do without holding it?

—Bohag Bihu Folk Song

Spring-time festivals that mark the onset of a new agricultural cycle are common all across India. Most spring-time festivals tend to be of the nature of folk festivals that differ from pan-Indian festivals such as Diwali. They are localised and their rituals and practices are rooted in vernacular belief systems and local material cultures; reflecting tight links between everyday life and the landscapes people inhabit. As folk traditions they include expressive 'forms, processes and behaviours' that utilise or display face-to-face interactions and that 'serve as evidence of continuities and consistencies through time and space in human knowledge, thought, belief and feeling' (Georges and Jones 1995: 1). *Bohag Bihu* is the spring-time festival of Assam. It is one of the oldest festivals of the region and is celebrated by all communities and across social strata within the state.

Today it is recognised as a prominent symbol of Assamese cultural identity. Besides the rituals pertaining to agriculture, *Bohag Bihu* evokes much gaiety through an array of music and dance performances that are at the core of this festival's celebrations. In contemporary times, with increasing industrialisation and urbanisation across Assam, new and innovative ways of celebrating the festival that imbibe modern technology, cultural influences and incumbent social sentiments have emerged. The most striking is the impact on the *Bihu* dance that is one of the most prominent features of the *Bohag Bihu* festivities. Historically, the *Bihu* dance is linked to the rural and agricultural backdrop. In the urban cityscape the dance performance has been located onto a stage that has effected the dance's form and invested in it contemporary socio-cultural sentiments of the Assamese people.

This chapter originated from ethnographic fieldwork conducted in Guwahati, one of the largest cities in lower Assam, and its surrounding areas during Spring 2009. The fieldwork included participation in *Bohag Bihu* festivities. The chapter focuses on the effects of the transference of the *Bihu* dance from a rural landscape onto an urban context. To explicate the effects of the urban locations and viewing contexts upon the dance, this chapter utilises ethnographic filmmaker David MacDougall's concept of 'social aesthetics', whereby human environments are understood as 'culturally constructed', reflecting the play of 'historical, economic and political forces' (2006: 58).

The concept of social aesthetics provides a necessary framework through which the urban performances of the *Bihu* dance can be situated within a wider historical project pertaining to micro-nationalist politics in Assam. Following India's independence from British colonial rule in 1947, Assam and other parts of North-east India have witnessed the rise of micro-nationalism of varying intensities and demands ranging from armed aggression and separatism to sovereignty and cultural integration within the wider rubric of the Indian nation. The Indian State has responded by adopting a largely defence-based, political approach that is clearly devoid of ethnographic rigour that would facilitate cultural and historical understanding of the Assamese region, its people and their ways of living. Within the mainstream Indian imagination, Assam, as is India's North-east in general, is sparsely represented in any sophisticated terms beyond the most reductive notions of primitivism and tribalism or ethnic conflict. The Indian media lacks resources, sensitivity towards and understanding of the Assamese political and cultural positions.[2]

The equation between Assam and mainland India follows the line of micro-nationalist politics within macro-nationalist frameworks that Sanjib Baruah argues as being 'obviously quite problematic' in ideological and political terms (Baruah 1994: 650). Deriving from Benedict Anderson and Gaston Bachelard, Baruah holds that:

'[t]he politics of micronationalism is premised on a poetics about a homeland and its people. If nations and nationalities are 'imagined communities' it is a poetics that transforms the geography of an area into primal, home-like or sacred space and transforms a people into a collectivity with imagined ties of shared origins and kinship'.

(Baruah 1994: 652)

Micro-nationalist sentiments are not limited to obvious political platforms and actions alone. As sentiments shared by communities of people they permeate social life and go on to inform expressions of culture. In view of this, micro-nationalism can be seen as not simply a defective or dissenting political category, but a force that shapes the performance of politics and culture. It bears the capacity to recontextualise folk and cultural practices by investing in their performance popular, political tempers. In this chapter, I will specifically discuss that the *Bihu* dance as performed in urban landscapes of Assam reflects a varied sentiment towards Assamese culture that I hold is informed by the micro-nationalist politics of Assam, but is also crucially distinct from Assamese insurgent separatism.

As postcolonial critic Aijaz Ahmad reminds us that when the category of 'nationalism' is yoked together with 'culture' 'to produce the composite category of cultural nationalism', it is worthy to understand that culture being distinct from other superstructures such as the economy is 'most easily available for idealisation and theoretical slippage' (Ahmad 1992: 8). The encounter between folk culture and Assamese micro-nationalism is subtle and devoid of aggressive and violent fervour that has come to be stereotypically associated with Assamese nationalism across the board. By interpreting how micro-nationalism affects the performance of a folk form such as the *Bihu* dance, we are positioned to appreciate the cultural sentiments of the Assamese people that have remained largely obscured within mainland India's representations and discourse surrounding the region. This is a necessary move that disassembles Assamese cultural thought as being fully in line with separatism and through that deconstructs Assamese micro-nationalism as monolithic, unified and sweepingly aggressive.

Assamese insurgency has been equated with demands for nationhood perpetuating a sense of cultural disparity, bordering alienation towards the Assamese. The viability of Assam as a small nation – I use the term 'small nation' in terms relative to mainland India – is debated and contested within that state and consensus on the subject has not been forthcoming. It is in this context that the points of departure between Assamese micro-nationalism politically and culturally gain importance for they complicate our understanding of Assamese conceptions of nationhood and sovereignty, beyond the stereotypical and reductive understanding of the region.

The chapter commences with an introduction to the origins and rituals of the *Bohag Bihu* festival, and the folk significance of the *Bihu* dance as a way to provide a historical survey of the folk form. The discussion then delves into *Bihu* dance in urban Assam. This discussion derives from my fieldwork that entailed participation in *Bohag Bihu* festivities and observation of the disparities in the form of the *Bihu* dance as performed in the city context and semi-urban communities on the outskirts of Guwahati. The observation undertaken during the fieldwork focussed on the dance form, its movements, body formations and expressions of the dancers in different locations. The chapter uses these observations as a way to map the disparities in the performance of the *Bihu* dance in the rural context and urban landscapes. The aim of mapping these disparities is not to create a comparison privileging one form of the dance over the other, instead I argue that *Bihu* dance in urban Assamese society has a distinct aesthetic that has evolved in response to the urban landscapes and it is mobilised to assert the Assamese cultural identity that is itself not in the spirit of a binaristic opposition or separatism towards mainland India, but is more in the spirit of inclusiveness through competing and consequently diverse modes of cultural and folk expression within the 'national imagination'.

The *Bohag Bihu* festival of Assam

Assam is a state in India's north-eastern region that is linked to mainland India via a narrow corridor of land in north Bengal called the Chicken's Neck. The north-eastern region of India is largely hilly with plains on either side of the mighty Brahmaputra river, which figures prominently in the folklore and mythology of the region. Topographically, the hills in the North-east are low and rugged, and the entire region has some of the finest, most dense rainforests. Assam has been primarily an agricultural society known for producing tea, paddy and jute. Historically, the people of the North-east are considered closer in culture to South-east Asia including Myanmar and Thailand, than South Asia including the Indian subcontinent. The 'region's geographical and cultural proximity to South-east Asia is reflected in its ethnic composition, which can be divided broadly into three groups: the tribes inhabiting the hills and those living on the plains, and the non-tribal population on the plains.' (Sonwalkar 2004: 393) The tribal communities are further subdivided into subtribes, and the entire region enjoys a rich diversity in its languages, dialects and folk life. Though Christianity spread across the region during the colonial era as missionaries converted tribal communities; in Assam, Hinduism is the predominant religion. Hindu and Vedic thought intermixes with tribal ways of living to create the distinctive folk forms of Assam.

Bohag Bihu is one among three festivals linked to the annual agricultural cycle in Assam: the other two being *Kati Bihu* (autumn) and *Magh Bihu* (winter). Of the three, *Bohag Bihu* is the most widely celebrated. Eminent Assamese folklorist, Praphulladutta Goswami observes that the prominence of *Bohag Bihu* within Assamese cultural life can be attributed partly to its strong '*adivasi* (tribal) pull' and partly to the agricultural setting of the region that according to him, fashions the 'social temper' of the Assamese people (Goswami 2003: 4). The Vedic texts of India prescribe rites and rituals to understand and control the movements within the cosmos and of the natural elements on earth. In the context of a pastoral society such as in Assam, these prescriptions historically served to mediate human relationship with land. Farming communities that depended entirely on nature sought ways of understanding the cyclical processes and changing patterns of nature as a way to better perform agricultural activity. *Bohag Bihu* festivities of Assam are strongly rooted in Vedic prescriptions. Goswami points out that the rites of *Bohag Bihu* are linked to the ancient text, the *Aitareya Brahmana*. 'These rites were meant to control the movement of the sun and thus secure reproduction [from earth]' (Goswami 2003: 5).

The term *Bihu* derives from the Sanskrit term *Visuvan*, meaning an equinox. *Bohag Bihu* is associated with the Vernal Equinox and it spans a week of rites, rituals, performances and celebration. The first day of the festival, on the Vernal Equinox, is called *Garu Bihu* and is dedicated to the worship of cattle used in farming. Various rituals such as offering garlands made from seasonal vegetables, casting away old ropes and replacing them with new ones and bathing the cattle and offering them sweetmeats are conducted on this day. The day after *Garu Bihu* is *Manuh Bihu*, and it is meant for human celebration. On this day people offer respect to their elders and exchange gifts. Traditionally the gifts included hand-woven Assamese outfits such as *mekhela-chaddor* (for women), *dhuti* (for men) and the *gamocha* – an intricately woven towel. In contemporary times, particularly in urban areas, gifts include Western clothing and the *gamocha* – that is a prominent symbol of Assamese cultural identity. On the third day of *Bihu*, congregational prayers are held in the community worship area of the village or city. There is no caste or class restriction within these spaces. This points towards the non-hierarchical nature of the *Bihu* festivities and accounts for their widespread popularity. The *Bihu* dance is performed from the fourth day of the festival. This is the most striking feature of the *Bohag Bihu* celebrations and is identified as a principle symbol of Assamese cultural life.

The *Bihu* dance

> As a woman embraces her lover, so may the earth take the seed of the rice into her womb.
>
> (Assamese Folk Song)

Spring gestures fertility. Within the Assamese folk worldview spring is seen as arousing passion. The *Bohag Bihu* festival, particularly the *Bihu* dances emulate this seasonal spirit – evoking and celebrating fertility and passion. Within the Assamese folk imagination, the earth is considered as mother and the sky as father. When the skies burst forth with monsoon showers, the seeds implanted in the earth mother's womb fertilise, producing a new crop that ensures the prosperity and well-being of the community. There are no historical records to exactly date and determine how old the *Bohag Bihu* festival is, but some ninth-century sculptures have been found in the Tezpur and Darrang districts of Assam that depict a dance which resembles the *Bihu* dance. Goswami holds that the *Bihu* dance is associated with some ancient springtime fertility cults (Goswami 2003: 38). Traditionally, the local farming community performed the *Bihu* dance in the open air in agricultural fields, bamboo groves, forests and on river-banks.

The *Bihu* dance, unlike the 'classical' dances of India, is not underpinned by a philosophical basis that venerates spiritual experience or the encounter with the Divine. Goswami states that:

> The *Bihu* dances are held in a reverential attitude, only the seasonal influence lending them a colour of comparative freedom. For Spring is also the period of mating. Underlying the whole festival is the desire for the welfare of the community, beasts and crops. That it is a sort of fertility cult is evidenced in the prayers offered by some of the Adivasis [tribals], though the Assamese themselves seem to have lost the original significance of this annual festival.
>
> (Goswami 2003: 40)

The *Bihu* dance is erotic with strikingly sharp and angular movements. It is performed by groups of young men and women who evoke fertility in relation to both land and humans. Men and women sing in altering turns, responding to one another. In earlier times, *Bihu* songs and dances were principally courtship dances that spilled into forests and fields. The songs reflect a principally pastoral sensibility and their themes include longing, anxiety of separation from one's lover and erotic love-play between lovers. Goswami qualifies that:

> The love depicted in folksongs is not normally the same thing as the spiritual exaltation and sublimation which the experience suggests in higher forms of culture. Its spontaneousness and artlessness are conditioned by the seasonal changes and the physical environments in which the people have their being.
>
> (Goswami 2003: 53)

In the *Bihu* dance, rhythm builds with repetition. The performers start by slowly walking into the performance space. The men commence by playing musical instruments including drums, horn-pipes and flutes. The women start by placing their hands just above their hips, palms facing outwards. The two hands are positioned in such a way that they form an inverted triangular shape. This resonates with the inverted triangle of Tantra Hindu worship practices where the shape is a fertility symbol representing the female reproductive organs.

As the music commences the women start to sway, bending slightly forward from the waist. They gradually open out their shoulders and spread their legs slightly apart – forming the principal posture for movement of the *Bihu* dance. Some of the movement sequences of the dance involve standing in posture and swaying sideways. As the music picks up in tempo the women thrust out their breasts and pelvis in alternation, synchronised with the rhythms of the music. As the tempo rises further, women may introduce a circular rotation standing in the same spot. Sometimes men and women form lines facing each other by clasping their necks or waists. In more advanced sequences of the dance, men and women pair up as couples at the centre of the performance space and perform gestures of copulation using their hands.

Since *Bohag Bihu* is linked to ancient fertility cults, the *Bihu* dance bears connotations of magic for rain to ensure the fertility of fields and humans. The music of horn-pipes and drums is held as replicating the sounds of rain-bearing clouds that serves to beckon actual rain. The abdominal and pelvic movements performed by the women in the *Bihu* dance are linked with sexual efficiency. As the music gains in rhythm and the women's movements of the pelvis and abdomen intensify and become more vigorous, a sense of ferocity emerges from the dance, through which the human body evokes and mediates the union of sky and earth, as well as getting itself sexually aroused.

There is historical evidence that the *Bihu* dance got socially looked down upon, particularly during colonial times when the performance's explicit erotics clearly conflicted with the Victorian worldview and its take on sexuality. The *Bihu* dance was affected and policed by this worldview. In contemporary times, the *Bihu* dance performance has assumed varied cultural meanings – those that exceed its origins as a dance to celebrate fertility and sexuality. The landscapes where it is performed play crucially upon how it is perceived, understood and performed. The next section discusses the performance of *Bihu* dance outside the pastoral landscape, in an urban context.

Bihu in the urban landscapes

Assamese urban landscapes arose steadily with the introduction of modernity during colonialism and its escalation after India's independence. The cities of Assam such as Guwahati, Dispur and Tezpur are linked to the rise of modern professions related to industry, tea export and services such as governmental administration and education. On account of the density of population in cities, the *Bohag Bihu* festivities here are conducted on a much larger scale than in the rural context – the magnitude only amplified by the use of modern technologies including advanced sounds systems and cameras. The celebrations are organised by local community bodies in the form of week-long cultural programmes. These cultural programmes are held in public spaces such as sports grounds that are centrally located and easily accessible. They are part of a fairground set-up including small stalls and shops that sell food, sweets, toys, music and consumer goods such as mobile phones. It was in a cultural programme in 1962 held at the Lataxil field in Guwahati that the *Bihu* dance was for the first time performed on a stage. Over the years, the cultural programmes have gained in popularity and expanded so that today they are financed through donations as well as corporate sponsorships.

The celebration of the *Bohag Bihu* festival in cities is primarily symbolic – serving to foster community and preserve people's links with their folk traditions as most urban populations have familial links with rural Assam. Alongside the *Bihu* dance the programme features musical competitions for children and adults, recitals by prominent Assamese artists and performers such as Bhupen Hazarika and a range of classical Indian and folk dances and performances such as Bharatanatyam and Kalbeliya. On these occasions, the *Bihu* dances have developed a form and vocabulary that displays variations from the *Bihu* dance of the rural/agricultural context. This calls up David MacDougall's idea that human life bears an 'aesthetic dimension' expressed in the environments people create around themselves. MacDougall states that human environments:

> [...] reflect historical, economic, and political forces, but also aesthetic judgments that directly affect how people live and the decisions they make. Human life thus has an aesthetic dimension expressed in the environments people create around themselves. In many cases, these settings – whether they be rural, urban, or institutional – provide islands of continuity in what is often a changing and hybrid existence, permeated by other forces.
>
> (MacDougall 2006: 58)

Bohag Bihu in the urban context has developed in response to the rhythms and dynamics of modern, city-based living and itself contributes to the specific aesthetics of the urban Assamese experience of culture and landscape.

The festivities witnessed by the researcher in Guwahati took place in an open ground including a stage a few feet high with seating arrangements facing it. Prominent social figures, visitors and a largely middle-class audience occupied the seating area that was barricaded. Members of the working-class audience sat either at the back or gathered on the sides of the seating area. In the urban context, it is common practice for stage backdrops to be decorated using local and folk materials with the intent to evoke the Assamese rural landscape. Usually a stage backdrop is a hand-painted scenography that includes prominent symbols linked to the landscape such as the low hills of Assam, wildlife, material culture artefacts such as *gamochas* and *sarais*. These scenographies tend to privilege the rural landscape as a way of evoking the landscape in which the *Bihu* dance is rooted, albeit in a nostalgic and romanticised gesture.

Since India's independence, *Bihu* dance groups and companies have emerged across Assam. These include local youth mostly from semi-rural and rural areas who train in the dance and during the festive season tour across cities and villages, performing on invitation as well as participating in *Bihu* dance competitions. The dance competitions are organised by local committees and offer winners prizes in cash or kind that serve to support the dance group's activities. The introduction of *Bihu* dance competitions has instilled the element of choreography and rehearsal in the *Bihu* dance performance, reducing spontaneity – that is at the heart of the *Bihu* dance as an agrarian folk form.

On stage, the performers either deploy the formation of vertical lines facing each other, or more commonly, horizontal lines where men stand at the back playing musical instruments and singing into microphones, while women are in the front to dance. Though the *Bihu* dance on stage is performed principally using linear formations, the choreographies do include short sequences when movements are performed in a circular formation. This is in sharp contrast to *Bihu* dance in the agricultural context where the performance takes place in circular or semi circular formations. There the *Bihu* dance is coextensive of agricultural activity and a circle comes about spontaneously when farming communities congregate to participate in the dance. Men and women then take turns and dance within this formation surrounded by the cheering onlookers. Within this circular formation the performer and viewer are not two distinct entities and there is no privileged viewing position.

Performing on stage institutes an emphasis on frontality as the performers directly face the audience. Frontal performance facilitates visual identification and display of the dance to an audience that is not inherently conversant with the vocabulary and meanings of the *Bihu* dance. In the urban context, display and exteriority are emphasised and the dynamic has shifted away from small community-based intimacy and interiority to public performance. As a consequence, the range of gestures and movements have been reduced to those most commonly associated, visually with the *Bihu* form. These form the basic vocabulary of an urban *Bihu* and are repeated within the choreographies. In recent years, the emphasis on frontality has been heightened with increasing media exposure of the *Bohag Bihu* cultural programmes as numerous local television channels provide live coverage. The visual regime of live television coverage requires multiplicity of image magnifications ranging from long shots that establish the stage space and location of the *Bohag Bihu* programme, to mid-shots that focus on groups of dancers and finally tight close-ups fragmenting and focussing on individual faces, hand gestures and footwork. Frontality during performance, exaggerated facial expressions, gestures and movements form a repertoire through which the *Bihu* dancers respond to the presence of cameras and the visualities they engender.

The stage space is physically, spatially and sensorially restrictive as compared with the open fields or riversides where the *Bihu* dance originated. The interaction between the male and female performers is reduced because they are now principally facing the audience rather than each other during the dance; and further because there are fewer instances in the actual choreographies when male and female performers freely deploy the erotic gestures of the *Bihu* dance. This has come about due to the policing of the form which began in the colonial era and continues now into a postcolonial context where public display of intimacy is socially restricted. At best, male and female performers now reference the erotic and flirtatious dimensions of the dance through small gestures of hands, eye contact or the occasional thrusting of torsos in movement.

In contrast with *Bihu* dance performances on stage, semi-urban localities on the outskirts of large cities have started to perform the *Bihu* dance in open spaces such as fields and grounds. Usually the dance is conducted in a large circular area demarcated by a low boundary line made of ropes and bamboo sticks. The audience is mostly working-class and surrounds the boundary line, either sitting casually or standing. This performance is underpinned by a sentiment to take the *Bihu* dance back onto the earth. Since these dances are performed in a circular space, they allow for more versatility in dance choreography – allowing for varied possibilities for formations and contact between the performers. The dance performance is thus more dynamic and vigorous. During the dances witnessed by the researcher, groups of men and women performed sequences by halting at different points along the circumference of the circle, allowing for closer engagement with a wider cross-section of the audience and facilitating a deeper sensorial viewing experience.

Within the micro-nationalist context

The transference of the *Bihu* dance from the agricultural landscape onto the urban stage is principally motivated by the need to make *Bohag Bihu* accessible to urban audiences whose social life may not be fully determined by the farming calendar but whose cultural heritage bears links to the farm-based folk traditions and practices of Assam. Urban *Bohag Bihu* celebrations serve to foster community and are underpinned by a nostalgia for the rural past. No longer primarily ritualistic in terms of agricultural links, *Bohag Bihu* festivities are entwined with the dynamics of cultural identity formation within the micro-nationalist context of Assam, serving to symbolise and evoke Assamese folk culture as a way to define and assert Assamese identity within the wider rubric of modern nationhood. The urban *Bohag Bihu* festivities have mobilised new social-spatial dimensions and index contemporary social sentiments within Assam.

In his discussion, David MacDougall emphasises that 'social aesthetics' consists 'not so much in a list of ingredients as a complex, whose interrelations as a totality (as in gastronomy) are as important as their individual effects' (MacDougall 2006: 98). Further, MacDougall qualifies that aesthetics in the social context has:

> [...] little to do with notions of beauty or art, but rather with a much wider range of culturally patterned sensory experience. It is thus not 'beauty-aesthetics' in the Kantian sense. Nor does it here imply the *valuation* of sensory experience (as in European

aesthetics), except as this bears upon the ability of people to determine what is familiar or unfamiliar.

(MacDougall 2006: 98)

Bohag Bihu festivities in urban Assam are evocative of rural Assamese life and landscape – coinciding with the element of familiarity that MacDougall raises. *Bohag Bihu* programmes particularly serve as interfaces for Assamese children and youth to engage with their 'traditions'. The *Bihu* dances are key visual exemplars of Assamese culture and have in the urban context come to symbolise Assamese cultural identity that is at once 'modern' and rooted in the Assamese landscape and way of life. These urban *Bihu* dances being choreographed rather than spontaneous, privileging linear formations to meet the spatial constraints of the stage, and including ossified gestures performed with an emphasis on frontality in a media-based context – differ significantly from the folk form of the agricultural context. On the stage, the *Bihu* dance evokes specific visual and sensory registers that arise as the dance form responds to the urban backdrop and the requirements that it engenders.

Despite the variations between the rural and urban *Bihu* dance forms, the situation of the *Bihu* dance in a cultural programme alongside other Indian classical dances is of significance to extend understanding of the cultural elements underpinning the micro-nationalist feelings of the Assamese people. This situation of the *Bihu* dance lends itself to be read as an expression of the people's sentiment for cultural inclusiveness within the wider rubric of India's cultural fabric thereby lending necessary complexity into the understanding of Assam's claims for separatism, sovereignty and small nationhood. In his discussion, Sanjib Baruah argues that micro-nationalisms such as in Assam '... have a purchase on the imagination of the peoples and produce higher-order obligations that compete with the obligations of national citizenship whose unquestioned primacy is best construed not as a given of social life, but as a project of the modern state. That does not mean that micro-nationalist demands are engaged in a zero-sum conflict with the state' (Baruah 1994: 652).

The *Bohag Bihu* festivities are representative of Assam's contemporary cultural fabric and will to preserve and assert Assamese cultural identity. This assertion of Assamese cultural identity may coincide with the micro-nationalist understanding of the cultural disparity between Assam and mainland India, but it does not necessarily coincide with a desire for breakaway nationhood or violence that is associated with the separatist movement. Performance of dances from other parts of India ranging from the classical Indian to *adivasi* (tribal) by non-Assamese artists and residents in Assam reflects the cultural diversity of post-independence Assamese society and in turn counters the summarily reductionist sentiments for ethnic cleansing often ascribed by conservative sections of the Assamese society as well as mainstream Indian media and popular imagination onto the entire movement in support of Assamese cultural resurgence. The cultural syncretism represented by the *Bohag Bihu* festivities exceeds the conflated disparities and binarisms posited by both the violent outfits within Assam on the one hand, and the defence establishment and mainstream media responding to that violence on behalf of the India state, on the other – thus unsettling the monolithic and homogenous terms through which Assam gets viewed and imagined within the Indian nationalist imagination. From a springtime fertility ritual dance to the urban stage, varied sentiments converge on the *Bihu* dance and situate in this folk form both traditional and modern cultural prerogatives.

Works cited

Ahmad, A. (1992), *In Theory: Classes, Nations, Literatures,* New Delhi: Oxford University Press.

Baruah, S. (1994), 'Ethnic Conflict as State – Society Struggle: The Poetics and Politics of Assamese Micro-Nationalism', in *Modern Asian Studies,* 28: 3, pp: 649–671.

Georges, R. A., and Jones, M. O. (1995), *Folkloristics: An Introduction,* Bloomington and Indianapolis: Indiana University Press.

Goswami, P. (2003), *Bohag Bihu of Assam and Bihu Songs,* Guwahati: Publication Board of Assam.

MacDougall, D. (2006), *The Corporeal Image: Film, Ethnography and the Senses,* Princeton and Oxford: Princeton University Press.

Sharma, A. (1999), *Assam: What is the Story?* Bachelor's dissertation submitted in partial fulfilment of BA (Hons.) Journalism, University of Delhi.

Sonwalkar, P. (2004), 'Mediating Otherness: India's English-language press and the Northeast', *Contemporary South Asia,* 13: 4, pp. 389–402.

Notes

1   *Muga* is a kind of dull-gold coloured silk, indigenous to Assam.
2   See Sonwalkar, 'Mediating Otherness: India's English-language Press and the Northeast', in *Contemporary South Asia,* 13: 4 (2004), pp. 389–440; and Sharma, *Assam: What is the Story?,* Bachelor's dissertation submitted in partial fulfilment of BA (Hons.) Journalism, University of Delhi (1999).

Index